CONNECTING
with
LIFE

Finding Nature *in an* Urban World

Martin Summer

Contents

Introduction 5

PART 1: A History of Nature and Humans 9

Chapter 1: The Beginning of Our Complicated Relationship 11

Chapter 2: Our Harmonious Relationship Changes Forever.................... 15

Chapter 3: The Rise of Farming and Science 19

PART 2: What's So Bad About Urban Living? 23

Chapter 4: How We Live Now: The Dangers of Becoming an Indoor
      Species 27

Chapter 5: Solutions: How Do We Get Outdoors More? 39

Chapter 6: Is Fresh Air a Thing of the Past? 45

Chapter 7: Solutions: Combatting Air Pollution 51

Chapter 8: Noise, Noise, Noise 55

Chapter 9: Solutions: Combatting Noise Pollution 61

Chapter 10: The Worrisome Case of the Missing Stars 67

Chapter 11: Solutions: Minimizing Light Pollution........................... 71

Chapter 12: The Shrinking Space in Our Growing Cities.................... 75

Chapter 13: Solutions: Combatting the Loss of Space 83

Chapter 14: How Fast Is Too Fast? 87

Chapter 15: Solutions: Combatting the Crazy Pace of Living.............. 91

PART 3: Finding the Balance Between Urban Living and Nature 95

Chapter 16: What Does Connecting With Nature Mean in Today's
      Urbanized World? 99

Chapter 17: Getting Mindful: Learning to Pay Attention.................... 105

Chapter 18: The Art of Using Our Senses: How to See......................... 111

Chapter 19: The Art of Using Our Senses: Seek the Sounds 115

Chapter 20: The Art of Using Our Senses: Smell the Roses (and Much More) 119

Chapter 21: The Art of Using Our Senses: Can You Taste Nature? 123

Chapter 22: The Art of Using Our Senses: Touch the World 127

Chapter 23: Other Senses Evoked in Nature 131

PART 4: Infusing Your Everyday Urban Life With Nature 137

Chapter 24: Can Technology and Nature Coexist? 141

Chapter 25: Designing a Nature-Friendly Home.. 151

Chapter 26: Stewardship Is More Important Than Ever Before................. 163

Conclusion... 171

About the Author.. 175

References 177

Introduction

ॐ

It took us over six hours in our rattling rented Toyota 4Runner to reach the best vantage point overlooking the Engilchek Glacier in eastern Kyrgyzstan at the border with China.

It was already dark when we arrived, so when we woke up the next day and saw what was right in front of us, we were speechless. A winding river separated us from the hilly plains morphing in the distance into a spectacular landscape. The glacier was massive, towering above already huge mountains below it. Its presence was almost unfathomable in the grassy open wild spaces under a warm summer sky. As cliché as it sounds, you do feel small in the presence of something so gargantuan and remote. Except for a handful of semi-nomadic families living in yurts sprinkled throughout the landscape and a small military base, there was nobody in the area. The closest town was a few hours away by car on the other side of a tall mountain pass with snow piled up even during the summer. Due east, there were no major human settlements for hundreds of kilometers. The tall, rugged mountains provided an impenetrable barrier.

Our ancestors would have laughed at us. To connect with wilderness, we traveled more than 4,000 kilometers (2,500 miles) by plane. Then we drove another 500 kilometers (310 miles). All this to enjoy a peaceful moment away from modern civilization. But where we come from—Poland, in highly urbanized Europe—such remote, untouched landscapes are rare.

The experience my girlfriend and I had in eastern Kyrgyzstan isn't anything out of the ordinary. People around the world seek to reconnect with their roots through exploring the wilderness. Some are blessed to have untouched areas right in their backyards. Others, such as us, need to travel long distances to get our fixes. In our everyday lives, we need to make do with nature of a more controlled kind.

We humans are drawn to the stillness of a forest. The rhythms of the ocean calm us. The majestic mountain landscapes make us feel awe. The wide open spaces of a grassy plain make us feel safe. Unfortunately, the world keeps urbanizing at a staggering pace. It's getting harder to connect with forms of life other than our fellow human beings.

There's no denying that our urban lives are better than the lives of our early ancestors. I, for one, wouldn't be able to live without a simple painkiller when I have a nasty headache. How about the Internet, cars, planes, and other incredible aspects of living in the modern, connected world? Technology is good for us, and it sure isn't nature's nemesis. It's understandable why even the most faithful nature lovers might prefer to live in a city. Urban areas offer many possibilities non-existent in rural areas:

- an abundance of career, education, and housing options,
- cultural and entertainment venues,
- public transportation,
- a range of shopping options,
- easier access to healthcare facilities,
- more chances of meeting new people,
- cross-pollination of ideas and subsequent rapid technological growth.

Cities can be incredible. But, as we've gained so much convenience, protection from the elements, and ease of living, we've also lost something. Human progress has gone hand in hand with increased pressure on wilderness areas, if not their outright disappearance. The ability to get away from everyone and enjoy an untouched, natural setting is a rare privilege for many modern humans. In many regions of the world—including Europe, the Middle East, large parts of Central and North America, East and South Asia—areas free of human footprint are non-existent or far and few between.[1] Increasing urbanization has cut us off from nature. Figuratively and literally. According to Yale School of Forestry and Environmental Studies, the global number of trees has fallen by approximately 46 percent since the start of human civilization.[2]

Nature has been the subject of a growing number of studies. They suggest it has an impact on our physical health[3] and how we perceive it.[4] Nature may also:

- decrease anxiety and help us think better,[5]
- improve our self-esteem and mood when engaging in an activity in the presence of nature,[6]
- offer psychological restoration.[7]

But you don't need me to cite hundreds of studies measuring the impact of nature on brain activity, cortisol levels, or a host of other bodily functions to know that nature is good for us. Many books have covered that truth. Don't get me wrong; scientific research into this topic is crucial. What I want to emphasize is that this isn't what this book is about (although I will refer to scientific research, too). Instead, I'll talk about what a city dwelling nature lover can do to stay sane in an urbanizing world. I'll provide ideas how to connect with nature when we have limited access to it. I'll explore what aspects of city living distance us from the natural world. I'll look at how to reduce their harmful impact on our well-being. We'll also learn how, through some simple choices, we can inject more nature than we realize into our cramped apartments.

The book aims to answer one big question: can we have it all, the convenience of a city and the nirvana of natural exposure?

I divided the book into four parts.

First, we'll talk about the history of human relationship with nature. This short overview will set the scene for the modern times. We'll discuss the challenges of urban living. Then we'll discover how they affect our physiological and mental health. We'll learn how we can deal with them to stay sane as nature lovers living in urban environments.

Next, we'll discuss how to find a compromise between our urban lifestyles and nature. We'll start with the key question of what nature means in today's urbanized world. Then we'll focus on the major threats to our health and well-being posed by our detachment from nature.

In the third part of the book, we'll look at simple everyday tools to reconnect with nature. You'll learn how to use your senses to deepen your connection with the environment.

In the last part of the book, I'll explore a plan for creating a modern life that balances urban life and nature. This will include how to best use technology. We'll take a look at how to design a nature-friendly home. We'll also learn how to take on the role of an environmental steward.

Your purchase helps the environment. I dedicate a part of royalties to support various environmental causes around the world. See the companion website at *www.MartinSummerAuthor.com* for more information on the initiatives I support. That's also where you'll find extra resources related to the topics mentioned in this book. You'll get a password to access them later in the book.

Now, let's delve into the backstory to learn how our relationship with nature has progressed and how we got to where we are today. When you finish reading the first part, you'll understand why we were so mesmerized by the wild open spaces of eastern Kyrgyzstan and the massive presence of the Engilchek Glacier. It will also become clear why humans are still so attracted to nature in all its forms, both spectacular as well as commonplace.

PART 1

A History of Nature and Humans

In the distant past, we used to bow to nature. Today, we give shape to it, control it, and decide who owns what piece of dirt and what's going to grow (or not) there.

In the modern world, we're more likely to talk about the human impact on the environment than the other way around. Global warming, destruction of ecosystems, and mass extinction are a few disgraceful consequences of ill-thought-out human activity. But for millions of years, the relationship was inverse: it was nature who bent us to its will. It shaped the everyday lives of our early ancestors. It impacted their evolution. It forced them to adapt as it changed. It was everything they knew and everything they needed.

The first great apes, *Pierolapithecus catalaunicus*, lived about 13 million years ago. The earliest *Homo* species emerged roughly 11 million years after. Both belonged to the natural environment as much as lions roaming the open savannahs, whales swimming in the oceans, or eagles soaring in the sky. Of course, there were biological and behavioral differences that have brought us to where we are today. But compared to modern times, our ancestors belonged to nature more than it belonged to them.

And then something happened. A change began that has lasted until today. We started adjusting nature to our needs. At first, on a tiny, insignificant scale that nonetheless marked a revolutionary milestone. To explore what happened in more detail, we need to hop into a time machine and teleport ourselves to the cradle of humankind.

CHAPTER 1

The Beginning of Our Complicated Relationship

ə▲

In December 1913, a worker supervised by German volcanologist and pale-ontologist Hans Reck found a bone at a site in what was then German East Africa. The bone led to the excavation of a human skeleton. It would be a major paleoanthropological breakthrough. It was the first discovery of an ancient human in the area, and one that Reck speculated was 150,000 years old.

Later studies showed it was in fact a body buried about 20,000 years ago. But the scene was set for other archaeologists, including Louis and Mary Leakey. Inspired by Reck, they uncovered in the same area fossils of ancient hominids and the earliest hominins. The former consists of all modern and extinct great apes. The latter consists of modern humans, extinct human species, and all our immediate ancestors.

The site where they worked—Olduvai Gorge, or modern-day northern Tanzania—is in the Eastern Serengeti. The Maasai call Serengeti the "Endless Plains". It's on those endless plains that we now find one of the most important paleoanthropological sites in the world. It's where we can get a glimpse into how early humans lived.

How early is "early?" Deposits at the site date back as far as 2.1 million years.[8] They include 1.8 million-year-old partial skeletons, skulls, and bones. The fossil discoveries provide evidence of likely dietary habits and behaviors, so different than the lives we lead today.

For example, *Paranthropus boisei*, an early hominin (but not our direct ancestor) likely ate mostly grasses and sedges (grass-like flowering plants).[9] The species had a powerful upper body and strong forearms used for climbing. Their bipedal and arboreal behaviors were crucial to surviving in its environment. *Paranthropus boisei* was the definition of raw strength. As Charles Musiba, a member of an international research team that excavated at Olduvai Gorge in 2010 and 2011, said, "It's unprecedented to find how strong this individual was. The stronger you are, the more adaptive you are."[10]

For the great ape ancestors 18 million years ago, raw strength defined their relationship with nature. The stronger you were, the better you fared. But while *Paranthropus boisei* stuck to the old ways, other early human species found another way to win the survival of the fittest game. The change started with *Australopithecus*, or *Kenyanthropus*, 3.3 million years ago and then early *Homo* 2.6 million years ago.

Rather than relying on brawn alone, they started manufacturing tools. That marked a significant turning point in our evolution. It was the moment when our relationship with nature began to change. Instead of using what our ancestors found in its natural form, they started shaping it to better suit their needs. They moved from sticks and stones to the first crude tools. They used them for woodworking, meat processing, digging up roots, and obtaining hide and fur. The first primitive shelters appeared. In 1971, at Olduvai Gorge, Mary Leakey found the oldest evidence of some form of hut structure. It was made of stone and tree branches. Those structures were temporary and a far cry from what we call "home" these days. Still, they were a great improvement over natural shelters such as nests in trees or caves.

Even with these huge breakthroughs, the lives of early humans were still dictated by nature. They were still hard. So hard that they're almost impossible to comprehend from the comforts of our air-conditioned homes. We have fridges full of food we didn't have to hunt for or gather ourselves. We relax in living rooms free from the dangers of predators and constant exposure to harsh weather conditions. Our ancestors had none of these luxuries.

Homo habilis began using tools about 1.8 million years ago to butcher and skin animals. Compared to only using bare hands or natural stones, it was an advancement like none before in history. Try to process meat—or even peel a potato—without any tools. It takes a lot of time and generates less than spectacular results unless you have razor-sharp nails. (By the way, a nail clipper is another underestimated benefit of modern civilization: before its invention people had to use small knives to trim their nails. Before that, early humans might have used their teeth, a rough stone or let the nails wear down naturally, which wasn't a pleasant sight.)

Gail M. Ashley and her colleagues from the Department of Earth and Planetary Sciences at Rutgers University spent years reconstructing a fine-scale model of an early human landscape. To create it, they used plant and other evidence collected at the site. When describing the lives of early humans, she said, "It was tough living. It was a very stressful life because they were in continual competition with carnivores for their food."[11]

Despite the discovery of stone tools, we were still at the mercy of nature. We were still very much a part of it on the same level as wild animals today. Our relationship with nature, even as it began to change with the invention of primitive tools, was still, for the most part, harmonious. It took another 800,000 years after *Homo habilis'* temporary settlement at Olduvai Gorge before our ancestors discovered how to control a tiny yet so powerful part of nature.

CHAPTER 2

Our Harmonious Relationship Changes Forever

&

The earliest known controlled use of fire took place in Wonderwerk ("miracle" in the Afrikaans language) Cave in South Africa, about a million years ago.[12] Before that, our ancestors relied on fire foraging. They collected resources like small animals that had been cooked in the aftermath of a lightning strike. The next step in their evolution was transporting fire from burned to unburned areas. Later, they learned how to start it themselves. As they improved their fire-starting abilities, they gained several important advantages. They could cook, which improved food digestibility. They could protect themselves, which reduced the danger posed by predators. They could keep themselves warm, which made a tough life a little bit easier. Sitting by the fire may have also sparked another remarkable turn: language development. To this day we seem to have the best conversations by the campfire, don't we?

Early humans were hunter-gatherers. They made temporary settlements as they moved in the search of food. For example, the Bushmen foraging in the Kalahari Desert moved every day during the rainy season. They were looking for edible greens during the day and slept in simple shelters at night. They would leave behind their campsites the following morning. When the dry season came, finding water was a critical task. That's when they built more stable huts around water sources.[13]

Controlled use of fire helped our ancestors survive in harsh environmental conditions when they were on the move. It didn't change one defining aspect of their lives, though. They were still very much at one with nature, spending their waking hours exposed to it and dependent on it. Everything they needed had to come straight from their surroundings. To get it, they couldn't spend the majority of their days in their caves. The lives of hunter-gatherers were the inverse of how we live today. We move from one shelter (our home) to another (our office) using a shelter on wheels (our car). We're rarely exposed to weather conditions. Often, we don't interact with a single sign of nature along the way. Consider how recent a change this is, too. According to the *Cambridge Encyclopedia of Hunters and Gatherers*, hunting and gathering occupies at least 90 percent of human history.[14] As a species, we're only beginning to learn a new way of living.

The discovery of fire wasn't an innocent skill with minor impact on the rest of nature. It was a steppingstone to humans separating themselves from the environment, if not positioning themselves above it. They were no longer another animal out on the plains. Now they could burn those plains and everything that lived on them on purpose. And they did so repeatedly for easier hunting and gathering.[15] The relative harmlessness of early human beings was gone. What was once one of many species announced its divorce from nature loud and clear. Whenever humans migrated into new parts of the world, a wave of extinctions of large animals followed. The migration caused biodiversity loss of enormous proportions.

When Neanderthals, Denisovans, and modern humans spread through Eurasia, mean body mass of mammals dropped by 50 percent. In Australia, the mammals became 10 times smaller. As *Homo sapiens* populating North America developed efficient long-range weapons, the mean mass of mammals fell by a factor of 13, from 98 to 7.6 kg (216 to 16.7 lbs).[16] To help you imagine how inconceivable of a change this was, think of it this way. If we drive to extinction all species currently at risk, the largest mammal on Earth in a few hundred years may be a domestic cow. And this would be the result of the mean body mass of mammals dropping by less than 50 percent. What happened in North America was of a factor of 13.

Hunter-gatherers and their new fiery talents had an unprecedented impact on the environment. They inflicted startling damage. But compared to modern humans, they were still on much friendlier terms with nature. Of course, small groups of ancient humans could do plenty of local damage. Overhunting and fire setting were destructive to the local environment. The effects compounded over hundreds of thousands of years and led to a global impact. But as troubling as they were as a species, one could argue they were still attuned to nature compared to what occurred about 10,000 years ago. This was when our modern history—and our progressing disconnection from nature—began in earnest.

CHAPTER 3

The Rise of Farming and Science

ક

Eight plant species called founder crops forever changed our relationship with nature. They were three cereals: emmer wheat, einkorn wheat, and barley; four pulses: lentil, pea, chickpea, and bitter vetch; and lastly, flax.

The cultivation of founder crops and the domestication of wild boars, sheep, and cattle formed the foundation of a new world. It was one in which human civilizations altered the natural environment on a previously unimaginable scale. More and more land was needed to supply the growing population. With each century, less and less land belonged to nature. Most humans turned their backs on the struggles of hunting and gathering out in the wild. They preferred to alter their surroundings to their benefit and convenience.

With the advancements in farming, small settlements grew into villages. Villages grew into cities. For the first time in history, some people—those born under the right circumstances—could live separated from the wilderness. Safe behind high city walls, they were more worried about their social status or the amount of metal coins in their pockets than about hungry predators lurking in the shadows or adverse weather conditions.

Not everyone lived an easy life away from the natural environment. In fact, most didn't. Farmers still lived off the land. Merchants were still exposed to elements as they traveled between settlements. Explorers could still travel to faraway places untouched by humans. And that's to name a few.

During the medieval period, people in the civilized world no longer lived as close to nature as the remaining hunter-gatherers. Compared to today, however, they were still exposed to it daily. If they were alive today, some would say that they were overexposed to the elements. Toiling away in the fields, they may have jumped at the opportunity to escape the hardships of nature. A warm bed in a high castle was more appealing than a cold hut by a primeval forest.

In a mere few thousand years, agriculture led to incredible human progress. It transformed us and our relationship with nature. This is in the wake of hundreds of thousands of years of no change in those relationships.

The Scientific Revolution altered our understanding of nature. Mathematics, physics, biology, chemistry, and astronomy have all contributed to major changes in how we lived. Newton's laws of motion and universal gravitation explained in his seminal *Principia* laid the foundation for the scientific method. These developments sparked interest in understanding the intricate mechanisms of the world. They further cemented human's status as a *de facto* owner of the world. Human was no longer one animal among many. It was an intelligent creature capable of transforming the entire globe with relative ease. It could even create new technology that could destroy in hours what nature had built in millennia.

As the centuries passed, more people moved to these ever-growing cities. In the pursuit of economic opportunity, they severed their ties with nature. But the driving forces behind migrations from the country to the city were dictated by necessity. There was no sudden animosity toward nature. People needed to put food on their tables, and cities offered more opportunities of doing so. There were also other factors at play. Parents wanted their children to live a better life than one spent toiling away in the fields. Those with controversial modern views (for the times) regarding, for example, feminism, sought refuge in a more progressive urban society. In the turbulent, war-torn times, those living in cities were often more protected than countryfolk, who were directly exposed to the worst of humankind.

The human migration over a mere 200 years happened on a massive scale. In 1800 less than 10 percent of the global population lived in urban areas. Each country has its own definition of what an "urban" area is, but it usually comes down to high population density and close-together buildings. In 1950, it was

30 percent. By 2018, that number had risen to 55 percent.[17] For the first time in history, we were now a predominantly city-dwelling species.

And that's how we got to where we are today. So many of us now live in sprawling cities, with small chunks of nature sprinkled here and there. We're struggling with problems unknown to our ancestors for almost the entire length of our presence on Earth. The ability to live safe lives shielded from the harsh conditions associated with living in the wilderness is a boon. Early humans couldn't have imagined it in their wildest dreams. But at the same time, it's a mixed blessing for the modern us.

There's no denying that we've benefited from our divorce from the natural world. While nature can be beautiful, it can also be inconvenient or deadly. We imagine our ancestors living simple lives in a perfect, untouched world. A wild, pristine world we might even long for. But viruses, bacteria, parasites, and mosquitos are as dangerous and deadly as lush Amazon rainforests, turquoise Caribbean waters, or koalas are gorgeous or cute. With full nature exposure, you get the whole package, warts and all. Except modern humans have altered it to their needs. Caribbean vacations? Of course. Dying from a tropical disease on your trip? No, thanks. Because of countless advancements, we don't have to deal with many of the unpleasant aspects of nature. We get to live longer and healthier lives.

Our lifespans are unimaginable to our ancestors. Based on Neolithic and Bronze Age data, the total life expectancy at birth wouldn't exceed 33 years.[18] This was partly due to high infant mortality and women dying at birth. The difference between our ancestors' and our modern lives is still staggering, though. Today, the world average is 72 years.[19]

We're better shielded from certain parts of the natural world, such as its dangers. I do like my Caribbean vacation without a dengue fever. But the other, more agreeable elements are missing in our lives. This deficit isn't a trivial First World problem. It doesn't apply to people living in developed countries alone. In fact, those living in poorer areas might struggle with access to nature even more. Budget-challenged countries can't afford the luxury of helping their residents get close to nature. Even in wealthy countries, the less affluent parts of cities are rarely beautified through nature.

But nature doesn't discern based on our socio-economic standing. The need to connect with nature is universal among humans, rich or poor, in Italy or in India, young or old, living in a metropolis or a minuscule village. I strive to encourage my friends and family to spend time in nature. Whether they live in a big city or in the countryside, their reaction is always the same. They *love* connecting with nature. I once convinced my parents (who live in the countryside) and one of their friends (who lives in a medium-sized city) to try winter swimming with me. We went to my favorite lake surrounded by a forest. To say they were exhilarated would be an understatement. It was connecting with nature that made the experience so rich.

According to biologist Edward O. Wilson's hypothesis popularized in his book *Biophilia*, humans have "the innate tendency to focus on life and lifelike processes." We seek connection with nature due to our evolutionary dependence on it. As Wilson poetically says, "To an extent still undervalued in philosophy and religion, our existence depends on this propensity, our spirit is woven from it, hope rises on its currents."

Even if today most humans live in urban areas and don't need to forage and hunt for food, we still need to connect with other forms of life to feel good. Examples abound. We spend a lot of money and time to travel to national parks and other wild areas. We love relaxing on the beach or in the water. We ski in the mountains. We take walks through forests. We take pictures of natural landscapes and wildlife. We hike in a variety of landscapes. Outdoor recreation is a huge industry generating more than 400 billions of dollars in the United States alone.[20] According to a report on the economics of biophilia, people will pay 58 percent more for property with a view of water. They will pay 127 percent more for a lakefront property. Good landscaping aesthetics coupled with large shade trees added an average of 7 percent to rental rates. Housing with excellent landscapes were priced 4 to 5 percent higher than similar houses with poor landscaping.[21]

Our craving for nature is evident in so many aspects of our lives. And yet we live in cities where it's difficult to connect with nature in our daily lives. It's a paradox that, as we've seen, is unique to our modern times.

Now that we've explored the past and acknowledged our present problem, let's dig into how today's world makes it hard to achieve this connection.

PART 2

What's So Bad About Urban Living?

With more than half of the world's population living in urban areas now and a projected two-thirds by 2050,[22] we are, beyond any doubt, an urban species. Humans can adapt to a wide variety of different natural environments. There are people living on the scorching hot plains of Serengeti. There are people in the humid rainforests of the Amazon. Our species inhabit the chilly Arctic tundra. They even live in the harsh, oxygen-deprived Himalayan mountains.

Living in a man-made environment, however, is new to us. How new, you might ask?

The emergence of anatomically modern humans happened about 200,000 to 300,000 years ago.[23] This is the beginning of our modern history. It hasn't changed much until the last several hundred years. It was particularly the period of the last 200 years when everything changed. We went from a tenth of people living in urban areas to well over a half in a mere 0.07 to 0.10 percent of our history.

Recent doesn't mean that it's wrong, though. The Internet, general anesthesia, and air conditioning are all new to us, too. That doesn't mean they're bad for us. We need to be aware of both their advantages as well as shortcomings. The

Internet connects people, but it also gives bad people new tools to harm others. General anesthesia saves us from indescribable pain, but wrongly administered it can lead to death. Air conditioning gives us thermal comfort, but it also increases the risk of infections.

Likewise, the population shift from rural to urban areas is in some respects good for our relationship with the environment. In other aspects, it's bad. Urban fertility rates are lower than rural fertility rates. This reduces population growth and its pressure on the environment. At the same time, urban populations consume more food, energy, and durable goods than rural populations.[24] With apartment buildings, high-rises, and smaller lots, cities are more space-efficient. At the same time, they encroach on natural habitats, causing habitat fragmentation or outright loss. According to a study on the impact of urban growth on biodiversity, the current pace of urban growth is equal to building a city the size of New York every six weeks.[25] These numbers don't offer much hope that future generations will be able to connect with other life forms and the natural world easily.

To make matters worse, there are also many ways in which living in a city affects our well-being. Urban areas may make our lives easier, for instance, but they disassociate us from the natural environment. This detachment isn't without consequence. Urban living with little to no access to nature is bad for us because we're genetically programmed to be in our natural environment. We need to be among other living things—not other humans alone.

If we turn our cities into places where no life outside of humans and an occasional tree exists, we will lose access to an essential part of our heritage and genetic programming. Who knows—we might be able to cope with new technological inventions. But I'd rather walk among real trees and see real wildlife than interact with virtual or artificial alternatives. This is why it's so important to understand why unbalanced urban living is bad for us. If we don't appreciate and embrace what other life forms have to offer and how crucial this relationship has been to us over the millennia, one day we'll lose this rich experience forever (and our sanity alongside it).

In this part of the book we'll discuss the biggest dangers of city living. We'll learn why they distance us from our roots and how this impact our health.

We'll address these challenges to learn to live closer to nature even in a bustling metropolis.

Unfortunately, urbanization has a far-reaching footprint. It extends well beyond the borders of a city. Even those not living in the biggest cities can suffer from a lack of connection with other life forms. That's why we'll also talk about less urbanized areas.

For easier reading, I discuss each problem in two chapters. The first provides an overview of the most severe effects of the discussed subject. The following chapter offers solutions. If you're looking for the how-to only, you can skip the overview chapter. I encourage you to take a look at description chapters, too. I did my best to describe each problem in a way that's not only educational, but also entertaining (I can't stand dry books!).

Let's begin with the biggest shift that has happened in recent years. It's caused by the growing numbers of urban population and the increasing convenience of city living. What is this problem? People spending the majority of their lives indoors.

CHAPTER 4

How We Live Now: The Dangers of Becoming an Indoor Species

કે

Each day, more than two thousand prisoners who live at the Wabash Valley Correctional Facility in Carlisle, Indiana are allowed to spend two hours outside. They describe this period as the most important time of their day, "keeping their minds right and their bodies strong." When asked how they would feel if their yard time was reduced to one hour a day, the inmates said they would feel sad, angry, and as if they were being tortured. Then the kicker is revealed: they learn that on average, children now spend only one hour a day outdoors.

This anecdote isn't a made-up story. It's from a real short film, with real inmates, produced for a marketing campaign ("Dirt is Good – Free the Children") by laundry brand Persil. You can watch this ad and access other resources on the dangers of urbanization on my website at *www.MartinSummerAuthor.com*. The password to access bonus content is "connecting."

How sad is it that modern kids spend less time outdoors than prisoners?

But then when we consider how little time law-abiding adults spend outside, it's no wonder that modern children don't have a good example to follow.[26]

According to research by World Health Organization and the U.S. Environmental Protection Agency, Americans and Europeans spend about 90 percent of time indoors. They divide their time between their homes, workplaces, schools, public places, and vehicles.[27, 28]

These numbers might be different for those who live in the countryside or in countries with more outdoorsy cultures. But there's no denying that urbanites, with their busy schedules, have little time to be outside. Even nature lovers who try to be outside as often as possible spend most time indoors.

If we sleep on average eight hours (the lucky ones among us, that is), that's already 33 percent of our days spent indoors. On any given weekday, most spend at least eight hours a day in an office (unless you work outdoors). This means that sleep and work alone already lead to two-thirds of our time spent indoors on an average weekday. When we calculate percentages for the entire week, assuming no work on weekends, we spend 57 percent of our time indoors just sleeping and working. Sadly, children probably spend the same amount of time, if not more, just sleeping and studying. That leaves us with 43 percent of our time each week to spend outside. But, of course, sleeping and working aren't the only two things we do indoors. We also engage in personal care activities. We commute, buy groceries, cook, eat, and perform various household activities. Even exercise now often means going to an indoor gym rather than being active outside. What little time we spend outdoors, we often don't even spend in nature. Instead, it's an uninspiring walk through an asphalted parking lot, a jog past a busy street, or mowing the lawn.

Why is spending time in our modern caves so bad? How does it detach us from nature?

Let's look at the main risks we face.

Indoor Air Pollution

The air inside buildings is often two to five times more polluted than the air outside.[29] Some of the delightful pollutants we breathe include:

- Biological pollutants—viruses, mold, bacteria, dead skin, and even droppings and body parts from cockroaches, rodents and other pests. We might like to connect with life in its richness of forms, but breathing body parts of pests doesn't sound like a good way to achieve it, does it?

- Carbon monoxide—unchecked levels of carbon monoxide in homes with improperly adjusted gas appliances can lead to death. Carbon monoxide is odorless and colorless, so it can kill you before you're even aware it's in your home.
- Lead—it's a naturally occurring element found in the air, soil, and water. Indoors, increased concentrations of lead come from, among others, deteriorating paint in older homes, pipes and plumbing materials.
- Nitrogen dioxide—homes with gas stoves, particularly when venting range hoods aren't used, are particularly exposed to excess levels. Homes with electric stoves can be exposed to high levels originating from local traffic.
- Pesticides—toxic insecticides and disinfectants can contribute to indoor air pollution. This also includes products used on lawns and gardens that you can track inside the house.
- Radon—the number one cause of lung cancer among non-smokers. It comes from the natural radioactive breakdown of uranium in soil, rock, and water. It gets into homes through cracks and holes in the foundation. If you live in an area where radon is a problem, test its levels and put in place reduction systems if necessary.
- Volatile organic compounds (VOCs)—emitted as gases from certain solids and liquids including composite wood products, paints, varnishes, wax, as well as household products used for cleaning, disinfecting, or degreasing. VOCs are found indoors in concentrations up to ten times higher than outdoors.

Indoor air pollutants can cause: irritation of the eyes, nose, and throat, headaches, dizziness, fatigue, respiratory diseases, heart disease, and even lung cancer.[30] Indoor air pollutants are also asthma triggers. According to a Finnish study, those living in damp homes had twice as high risk of asthma and a greater chance of repeated colds and skin allergies.[31] It's clear that the more time we spend indoors, the higher our risk of getting sick.

Nature lovers or not, we all live in modern dwellings and pay a price for the convenience they offer. The goal isn't the complete elimination of indoor pollutants, which would be impossible. It's their reduction, which we'll cover in the next chapter where we'll consider some solutions to help us enjoy more fresh air.

Increased Risk of Contracting Airborne Infections

That lovely flu you seem to get every winter is largely courtesy of spending increased time indoors. The virus is more stable at lower relative humidity,[32] which characterizes our modern air-conditioned caves. Moreover, in dry air, each cough and sneeze of an infected person is more dangerous. The particles from their noses and mouths break into smaller pieces in dry air compared to moist air. These smaller pieces can stay airborne for hours or even days. Yes, the frightening reality of spending a lot of time indoors is that each day we're breathing viruses spread by other people who were in the same room.[33]

There's some evidence that contact with nature may boost immune system through exposure to essential oils and common soil bacteria Mycobacterium vaccae. Consequently, nature-loving city dwellers are potentially more protected from the increased risk of infections when spending time indoors.[34]

Insufficient Natural Light Exposure

Unlike our ancestors, we often emerge from our caves only when it's dark. According to German professor of chronobiology Till Roenneberg, an average employee on an average workday spends a mere 15 minutes outdoors during the daylight hours.[35] It's easy to understand why. There's little time in the morning to take care of all the household chores, let alone go outdoors. With an average person working until five, they often get home at six or later. All daylight hours go by while they're in the office.

This troubling, unnatural tendency has a massive impact on many aspects of our lives. Humans have inner clocks called circadian rhythms that regulate our sleep-wake cycle. One of the main factors influencing them is the amount of natural light we get (or not).[36] When we fail to get natural light when the body expects it, our health suffers. This is what happens when we're locked during the day in a dim office.

When we expose ourselves to strong artificial light when the body doesn't expect it, our health also suffers. This is what happens when we watch TV or use our smartphones at night. For a good example of how this works on a more extreme level, hop on a plane, cross ten time zones, and see how well you can sleep for the next few days. Disturbances of the circadian rhythm can affect general health,[37] sleep quality and mood[38] as well as metabolism. Scientists are now investigating the impact of desynchronized body clocks on obesity and diabetes.[39]

Those with their circadian rhythms destabilized to the greatest extent— night-shift workers—have higher rates of cardiovascular disease, cancer, obesity, and diabetes.[40] Night shifts are unnatural. A meta-analysis by French chronobiologist Simon Folkard shows that as many as 97 percent of night-shift workers fail to completely adapt to their work pattern. Yes, you read it right. Almost every single night-shift worker struggles to adapt. To make matters worse, of this number, 75 percent don't adapt to their night shift at all.[41] In light of these findings (pun intended), we owe much respect to those who work at night and sacrifice their health for their professions.

Outdoor levels of light on a sunny day will help regulate the circadian clock in 30 minutes. The sad reality is that we're not exposed to even a fraction of these levels if we spend the entire day indoors. Typical light levels in our homes tend to be around 150 lux, while a recommended light level in an office is 500 lux. Lux is a measure of the intensity of light as perceived by the human eye. When you sit by a window on a cloudless day, you're exposed to about 1,000 lux. Away from the windows you might be exposed to as little as 25 to 50 lux.

And here's the kicker: when you're outside in full daylight but not direct sun, you're exposed to 10,752 lux. With the sun overhead, illuminance reaches up to 107,527 lux. That's 716 times more than when you're at home, 215 times more than in an office, and 107 more even than sitting by a window! Even on an overcast day, you're still exposed to 1,075 lux. The only exception is a very dark day when the light level is a pitiful 107 lux.[42] Other than that, our everyday indoor lights are no match for what nature has to offer. Yet, so many of us go days or weeks on end without sufficient exposure to this precious gift.

What about those who work outdoors?

According to the U.S. Bureau of Labor Statistics, 47 percent of jobs held by civilian workers require work outdoors at some point during the workday. However, the jobs most likely to require outdoor work include: construction and extraction occupations, protective services, installation, maintenance, and repair, and building and grounds cleaning and maintenance.[43] Except for protective services and some maintenance jobs, all those jobs involve urban settings, often with additional health risks. For example, construction workers are exposed to dust, chemicals, or outdoor air pollution. This makes even those working outdoors at a risk of not getting enough natural light or getting it at a high cost.

Insufficient Vitamin D and Sun Exposure

The human skin synthesizes vitamin D upon exposure to UVB radiation from sunlight. Glass absorbs UVB, which is why you can't get a sunburn—or vitamin D—when sitting by a window. Of course, in true modern human fashion we can take vitamin D supplements. We can also rely on a few dietary sources of the vitamin (including fortified foods) instead of spending more time outside. But the real thing works better. Vitamin D made in the skin lasts twice as long as vitamin D from the diet. Moreover, sunlight provides between five to ten extra photoproducts you can't get from the supplement. It also offers important positive psychological effects.[44] I'm not sure about you, but I take no pleasure from swallowing vitamin D. Meanwhile, spending time in the sun (intelligently, without getting sunburned) is one of my favorite pastimes.

As a person suffering from SAD (more on that later), I notice an immense change in my mood when it's sunny outside. When I meet new people, I like to ask the ones who moved from a cloudy area to a sunny one if their mood has changed. They all emphasize how massive of a difference it has made. Some dread coming back to their hometowns or home countries for more than a few days. In their new lives, they expose themselves to sun regularly and thrive because of that.

If you need any further proof how valuable (smart) sun exposure is, consider where most retirees head to. Florida, Mexico, Costa Rica, Spain, Greece, Portugal, and Italy top the lists of best places to retire. All of these places make it easy to spend time in the sun. That's not to say you can't be healthy when you live in a country with frequent dark skies. It does take more work and it is less rare to enjoy sunshine in such places. However, this only makes it more important to develop awareness of how little sun and vitamin D you get by spending too much time indoors.

Vitamin D is essential for bone health,[45] the immune system,[46] and physical performance.[47] That excess time spent indoors leads to a big health risk. City-dwelling nature lovers might not suffer from vitamin D deficiency as much as those less interested in nature. However, to get vitamin D naturally, we need to expose our bare skin (without sunscreen) to the sun while it's high in the sky, when UVB radiation can reach the ground. This is often when an average city dweller is in an office. As a result, a typical urbanite might only be able to expose themselves to the sun on the weekends. This might not be enough to achieve healthy levels of vitamin D. If this is you, take advantage of your lunch breaks to spend time in the sun. If not possible, supplements might be helpful.

Note that if you live in a temperate climate, you can't get vitamin D during the winter at all. That's because the sun's angle is too low to cause the skin to synthesize vitamin D. Supplementation (or frequent trips to warm climates if you can afford it) is thus essential, or you may end up deficient by spring.

Seasonal Affective Disorder

Seasonal Affective Disorder (SAD) is a condition caused by the reduction of sunlight in winter. It leads to depressive symptoms that get even worse when you spend too much time indoors. The prevalence of the condition depends on your location. In the U.S., 9.7 percent of people suffer from SAD in New Hampshire. Meanwhile, this number is only 1.4 percent in sunny Florida.[48] It affects about 6.1 percent of the entire U.S. population,[49] 2 to 6 percent of

Canada, about 8 percent of the United Kingdom,[50] and between 2 to 8 percent of the total population in Europe.[51] There's also Subsyndromal Seasonal Affective Disorder (sometimes called "winter blues"), which is a milder form of SAD. It affects 14.3 percent of the U.S. population, 15 percent of Canadians, and 21 percent of the UK population (I was unable to find data for the total European populations).

For those who suffer from this condition (including yours truly, who, at the moment of writing this is sitting by a SAD lamp on a dreary January morning), adequate light exposure is even more crucial to manage the symptoms and avoid debilitating winter sluggishness. Being a nature lover can help motivate those suffering from SAD to head outdoors even in adverse conditions. However, with decreased energy and reduced access to nature, this can be more challenging for an average city dweller (again, yours truly included). In the most extreme cases, SAD can lead to a cascade of negative effects, including severe depression.

Myopia

Spending too much time indoors is linked with what's referred to as the myopia epidemic. It's a dramatic increase in short-sightedness among teenagers and young adults around the world, most notably in East Asia. In China, up to 90 percent of teenagers and young adults have myopia—that's compared to a mere 10 to 20 percent 60 years ago. In highly urbanized countries of Hong Kong, Singapore, South Korea, and Taiwan, more than 80 percent of 20-year-olds suffer from near-sightedness. That's compared to 20 to 30 percent 60 years ago.[52] In the United States and Europe this number is about 50 percent, double what it was 50 years ago. Would our ancestors ever imagine a future in which over a half of the young population in some of the most prosperous countries in the world can't see well?

Researchers have found that the only environmental factor that was strongly associated with risk was time spent outdoors. Children who spent less time outside were at greater risk of developing myopia. Scientists controlled for physical activity. They found out that what seemed to matter most was the eye's exposure to bright light, regardless of the type of activity in which children participated outdoors. But as we've already learned from the short film shot at Wabash Valley Correctional Facility, an average child spends a mere hour outside. This shouldn't be a surprise that they start having health issues so early.

Nature-loving urbanites might be less at a risk of myopia if they spend their weekends—and any possible spare time, for that matter—outside. However, it's important to note that in dense cities, daily access to sunlight becomes a precious commodity. Walking down a city street shaded by skyscrapers might not expose our eyes to enough sunlight. As a person living in a medium-sized city, I'm always amazed at how dark the downtowns of big cities are. Sometimes even urban parks aren't enough as they're also surrounded by tall buildings.

In New York City, the plans to build super-tall, ultra-thin luxury apartment buildings around Central Park have created controversy because of the shadows they'll cause. Other major cities around the world struggling with space might soon face the same dilemma. The amount of natural light entering a house is already a big selling point in temperate or cold countries. Imagine how much worse it may get if our cities keep growing taller and taller, reducing the amount of sunlight for those who can't afford to live on the top floors. What sounds like a dystopian scenario is already a reality for some people.

Insufficient Physical Activity

Our ancestors moved every single day, often for hours on end. They hunted, gathered food, collected materials for a temporary shelter, or walked from one location to another. Some climbed trees, some dived to gather seafood, some ran and ran and ran until their prey fell, exhausted and overheated. It was a difficult life that even today's top athletes would find tiresome. Today, on some tough days, we don't even feel like moving from the couch to the fridge unless an irresistible treat awaits us there. A convenient life is addictive. Why move so much if you can have everything delivered to your home? It's easy to get stuck in a vicious cycle reinforced by popular passive indoor activities such as watching TV or browsing social media. In a battle between our self-discipline and our sofas, it's the latter that usually delivers a crushing win.

According to a report from the Centers for Disease Control and Prevention, only 22.9 percent of U.S. adults aged 18 to 64 met the guidelines for both aerobic and muscle-strengthening activities.[53] If you're curious about the official guidelines for exercise, it's a mere two and a half hours per week of moderate physical activity. Alternatively, it's 75 minutes per week of vigorous physical activity. That's in addition to muscle-strengthening activities two or more days per week.

To some, it might sound like much. But when you think about it, we're talking about three or four hours out of your entire week. And that's for an activity that has been proven to extend your life and make it better. I have friends who spend up to a few times more time playing video games than caring for their bodies. Isn't there something wrong with our balance of sedentary and active life?

Europeans don't fare better than Americans. Statistics from Europe show that 29.9 percent of the population aged 18 or over in the European Union spent at least two and a half hours per week doing physical activities. This included cycling as form of transportation, though, which is more prevalent in the EU than in the U.S.[54] In other words, 70% of Europeans fail to exercise enough. The statistics are undoubtedly similar for various countries across the world.

Cities can help their residents be more active with all the convenient places they offer to exercise, but they can also provide a distraction in the form of all their enticing indoor attractions (theaters, shopping malls, restaurants, bars, clubs, etc.). Moreover, those who do exercise often choose air-conditioned indoor gyms over parks. Thus, they miss out on the benefits of outdoor physical activity. In some sports, there's been a shift from more difficult to control outdoor environments to controlled indoor ones. Rock climbing is one such example. Initially performed only outside, indoor rock climbing on artificial walls in dusty climbing gyms has experienced meteoric growth. Many of my climbing friends exercise almost exclusively indoors. They get the benefits of exercise, but climbing on plastic doesn't provide the feeling of connection a true piece of rock offers.

The problem of spending too much time in our modern caves isn't limited to city living. Even those living in rural areas are often members of the indoor generation.

Freelance writer Hettie Harvey was tired of worrying about money, commuting, pollution, and crime in London. She decided to move to the countryside with her family. She wrote about her expectations in an article for The Telegraph: "Having done next to no exercise in years, and never having dropped below a size 12 since hitting puberty, I was also convinced that almost overnight I'd become super-fit and sylph-like with all the exercise and fresh air that we were going to be getting. Which sounds perfectly reasonable until you factor in having to get in the car to do anything, even just to buy a pint of milk. The reality is that I've never been less active in my life and am expanding steadily, day by day."[55]

Harvey is not an exception to the rule. A study on urban and rural adults of various socioeconomic backgrounds in the United States found that rural residents were least likely to meet physical activity recommendations. Meanwhile, suburban residents were most likely to meet them. One of the important factors was income.[56]

According to the researchers, the number of places available for exercise increased the likelihood of regular exercise. This would put urbanites at an advantage. They have access to well-lit sidewalks, walking and jogging trails, parks, and gyms. Those living in rural areas don't have the same convenience. This is most challenging if they live in flat, farming regions where nature is often even more sparse than in a big city.

But there's a caveat. While the lack of infrastructure might affect physical activity levels, it's also possible that those who live in the countryside get more exercise through occupational and domestic tasks rather than through leisure, which is what the study measured. When my parents moved from the city to the countryside, their physical activity levels increased primarily through new domestic tasks. Living by a forest, they took walks more often, too. However, their largest increase in exercise came through gardening, chopping wood, or working on various house improvement projects. You don't engage in any of these tasks when you live in a small apartment in the city.

There's no question that living by the beach, a forest, a lake, mountains, or any other wilderness area helps. It's a more inspiring setting to get out, get active, and get some fresh air. I did find it easier to spend more time outdoors when I lived in sunny countries, close to the ocean or surrounded by nature. But whether you live in a city apartment or a rural house, you can still spend entire days indoors. Both city and rural residents may spend entire days browsing the internet, watching TV, playing video games, or engaging in other activities in the safety of their modern caves. In the end, it's us, not the environment, who decide how much time we spend indoors and outdoors.

Overcoming the allures of indoor living may help us live healthier and happier lives. So, how do we deal with the dangers of indoor living and make our lives resemble the lives of our ancestors a little bit more?

CHAPTER 5

Solutions: How Do We Get Outdoors More?

ॐ

Our modern, urbanized lives have forced us into becoming indoor species. When compared to the lives of our ancestors, we're not only detached from nature, but from the general outdoor world, too. This is not necessarily a bad tendency. Few if any things are black and white when we talk about how different our lives are than the lives led by humans who didn't live in an urbanized world.

We're safer, more productive, and more comfortable when we can protect ourselves from the elements. There's no doubt that it's good to have a roof over your head. At the same time, the more time we spend outside, the better it is for our well-being. As discussed already, we need natural light, fresh air, and physical activity to thrive. It's our inner wiring, an internal mechanism that makes us feel good each time we spend time outside. But it's neither practical nor sensible to expect that an average person, particularly someone living in an extremely cold or hot climate, can somehow "rebel" against the system and spend most of their time outside. When weather conditions are adverse, life without our modern dwellings is *hard*. Even those who spend extended time away from civilization can appreciate the benefits of indoor living. Maybe they can even appreciate them more than a faithful city dweller. I sure did after coming back home on the brink of hypothermia after three miserable days camping in cold, wet conditions.

The goal is to find balance between indoor and outdoor living so we can live a little closer to nature *without* losing the benefits of indoor living. A good starting point is to develop awareness of what your current balance is like. Research suggests that people underestimate how much time they spend indoors.[57] You can track your activities for a week to estimate how much time you spend indoors versus outdoors. These numbers will differ depending on the season, unless you live in a climate with little variance.

For example, I'm embarrassed to admit that during an average winter week in Poland I usually spend no more than ten hours outdoors. That means I spend a mere 6 percent of my time outside. But hey, I have good excuses—I hate cold, overcast weather and feel sad looking at all the leafless trees. On a more serious note, I should do better than that and am trying to correct it. Meanwhile, during an average summer week, I usually spend at least 30 to 40 hours outdoors. That's a much more respectable 18 to 24 percent of my time spent outside. If I'm on extended vacation out in nature, these numbers might be more than double that.

Once you know your ratio of time spent indoors to outdoors, you can commit to shifting the balance. Every percentage counts! One way to achieve this with little effort is to identify which everyday activities don't require you to be indoors. For example, you can have lunch outdoors, even if it means sitting on a bench in front of the office building. You can have a call when on a walk in a park. If you're reading a book, read it outside, on a terrace, balcony, or under a tree. If you're going to a restaurant, dine al fresco whenever possible and comfortable. Consider commuting by bike if it's practical where you live. You might not consider it "proper" nature exposure. But you're still getting outside, soaking up some sunshine and (hopefully) getting some fresh air. This also strengthens our connection with the richness of life as we escape the stale air of our dark caves.

Weekends offer the possibility of making up for the little time you spent outside during the week. Don't waste them. Day or weekend trips to destinations close to your city don't have to be expensive. Having a picnic in a park costs you nothing other than money for groceries you'd buy anyway. These simple activities might be even cheaper than going shopping, eating out, or finding other ways to spend money. Indoor venues excel at somehow making money disappear out of our wallets, don't they?

If you prefer multi-day nature outings, don't fall victim to the trap of waiting months for your next trip. Nearby nature, even close to or within urban areas, or even in your backyard, is still better than staying at home and watching TV. I prefer spending time in wilder areas, too, but with the limits of time and money it's better to take what's available than nothing at all.

Taking up a sport you can practice outside is another good idea. And again, it doesn't have to be an activity you practice in pristine, wild nature. Calisthenics (bodyweight exercises, usually involving pull-up bars and similar equipment) is one way I get regular natural light exposure while living in a city. I could practice this activity indoors, but doing it outside, rain or shine, helps me get some natural light exposure and toughen up a little when the conditions aren't favorable. If outdoor sports aren't possible, enrich the experience of your indoor workouts by listening to natural sounds. You can also watch natural landscapes. Visualize that instead of simply exercising on a stationary bike, you're riding through a picturesque setting.

The outdoor activities you engage in don't have to be strenuous or extreme. Consider photography, even if it's taking pictures of your city's nature or the little inhabitants of your backyard. Try your hand at gardening, even if it means caring for a few plants on your small balcony. Visit street fairs or farmers' markets or maybe even drive to a farm that sells produce directly. Buying produce straight from a person who grew it also makes us connect with nature, particularly when you compare it to the lifeless experience of getting your fruits and veggies from a supermarket.

Another way to get motivated to spend more time outdoors is to get your friends involved. Instead of meeting in a bar, go for a hike, rent a kayak, or take a walk in a park. Besides getting natural light, you'll also create memorable experiences. Let's be honest; you'll forget another bar visit in a matter of days. Meanwhile, stand up paddle boarding down the city river will stay a vivid memory for years to come. Of course, there's nothing wrong with indoor leisure time. Just make sure there's a balance between time spent indoors and outside.

Speaking of spending time indoors, let's now address the big problem of indoor pollutants. Get more fresh air through opening the windows a few times a day to air out the house or office. This simple habit can do wonders to the indoor air quality. Avoid doing it on days with extreme outdoor pollution, though. Other solutions to reduce indoor pollution levels include not smoking indoors, minimizing clutter that attracts dust and vacuuming often. Consider using natural cleaning supplies in contrast to harsh chemicals that give off harmful fumes. Air purifiers can also be helpful if you struggle with low indoor air quality. Contrary to popular belief, indoor plants don't make a difference in the amount of volatile organic compounds polluting indoor air unless you stuff between ten and 1,000 plants per ten square foot (one square meter).[58] As a side note, this doesn't mean that indoor plants are useless. They just aren't efficient at purifying air compared to ventilating the house.

Another easy action that will help diminish the negative impact of indoor living is to let in as much daylight as possible. Unless necessary, don't use shades, curtains, drapes, or blinds. Keep your windows clean and sit as close to them as possible. When at home, spend most of your time in the brightest room. Maximizing natural light exposure will bring your daily rhythm a little closer to that of our ancestors.

Since very overcast days fail to provide enough natural light, if you suffer from Seasonal Affective Disorder, consider investing in a bright white, full-spectrum SAD lamp. The most effective lamps provide light at 10,000 lux when they're one to two feet (30 to 60 cm) away. The therapy is effective with 30 to 60 minutes of daily exposure.[59] Position your lamp in front of you, but don't stare at it directly (think of it as the sun).

I've been using a SAD lamp for several years. I turn it on in the morning for up to two to three hours while I work. I don't suffer from side effects of overuse, but some people may get headaches or feel nauseous. It's an invaluable aid to survive the darkest months with little sunlight. When spring comes and sunshine is more abundant, I reduce my use of the lamp until I don't need to use it anymore and can rely on the good old sun in the sky.

To sum up, here are the key actions to take (you'll find this quick summary after every chapter with solutions):

&- Develop awareness of what your current balance between indoor and outdoor living is like. Then commit to shifting the balance in favor of outdoor living through everyday choices. Have lunch outdoors. Take calls while on a walk in a park. Commute by bike, etc.

- Take advantage of weekends to spend more time outside. Choose outdoor activities over indoor venues.

- Think how you can spend time outside every day over waiting for multi-day trips. One way to do so is through participating in outdoor sports. This can be something as simple as taking a brief walk every day or activities including photography and gardening.

- Organize fun outdoor activities for your friends instead of defaulting to spending time in a bar, night club, or a similar indoor venue.

- To improve indoor air quality where you spend most time, air out your living space and your office regularly.

- Vacuum frequently.

- De-clutter regularly to avoid dust build-up.

- Use natural cleaning supplies that don't give off harmful fumes contributing to the low indoor air quality.

- Consider investing in an air purifier.

- To avoid the negative effects of insufficient light exposure, let in daylight as much as possible and sit close to the windows.

- During the winter, if you're struggling with Seasonal Affective Disorder (SAD) or winter blues, use a bright white, full-spectrum SAD lamp.

CHAPTER 6

Is Fresh Air a Thing of the Past?

⁂

When the coronavirus outbreak spiraled in India in March 2020, the residents of New Delhi, the world's most polluted capital city, were ordered to stay at home to prevent the spread of the virus. A huge reduction in traffic improved the Air Quality Index (AQI) immediately. It dropped from average 161 (considered "unhealthy") to 93 (considered "moderate"). Consider that even with the country's activity reduced to the minimum, the air quality was still well above levels considered "good" (below 50). Yet, for the city's residents used to unhealthy levels on most days, the improvement was massive.

Skyscrapers were no longer shrouded in smog. Stars were visible in the sky. As retired sea captain Francis Braganza, whose wife suffers from chronic breathing problems caused by pollution, said, "We went for a walk and my wife found that breathing was easier."[60]

Many countries around the world that put in place similar measures experienced similar air quality improvements. But not for long. As the restrictions lessened, the air quality decreased again.

According to the World Health Organization (WHO), air pollution is now the world's largest single environmental health risk. Each year it kills millions of people around the world[61], with global estimates as high as 8.9 million deaths.[62] We might no longer be killed by predators or exposed to the elements but as we made our lives more convenient, we've created another deadly problem.

One of the scientists behind a study estimating the mortality caused by air pollution, Thomas Münzel at the University Medical Centre Mainz in Germany, puts the number of deaths into perspective by pointing out that air pollution causes more deaths a year than tobacco smoking.[63] Unfortunately, while you can decide not to smoke, you can't decide not to breathe.

The WHO warns that more than 80 percent of people living in urban areas that track air pollution are exposed to air quality levels that exceed the acceptable limits. Poorer countries are more affected than wealthier countries. The standards there are often less stringent. The public is less educated. The local inhabitants can't afford more eco-friendly solutions to heat or cool their homes. 98 percent of cities in low- and middle-income countries with more than 100,000 inhabitants don't meet the guidelines. In high-income countries the situation is better (but still grave) with 56 percent of cities failing to meet the standards.[64]

In some cities—particularly in India—the problem is so bad that schools are shut down during periods of extreme pollution.[65] Guidelines to deal with high levels of air pollution in Delhi sound like they are taken from a post-apocalyptic movie. Firstpost, an Indian news and media website, says: "It is advised that a person covers their face, wears bandanas, glasses, hand gloves and focuses on protective clothing before heading out in open."[66]

Long-term health effects of air pollution include: heart disease, stroke, chronic obstructive pulmonary disease, lung cancer, and respiratory infections.[67] Short-term effects include: difficulty in breathing, coughing, wheezing, and asthma. Worsened symptoms of existing respiratory and heart conditions are also common. The human body wasn't made to breathe the toxic air of our modern cities.

Those nature lovers who often spend time in wild areas might give their lungs a break during their trips. Unfortunately, when they're back in their cities, they suffer like everyone else. Unlike dealing with the problem of indoor living that we can address individually, there's little a single resident can do to improve the air quality of the city in which they live. There are some solutions, which we'll discuss in the next chapter.

Are rural areas better if you want to breathe fresh air?

In the U.S., according to the Centers for Disease Control and Prevention, air quality improves as areas become more rural. Compared to large metropolitan cities, rural areas get over ten times fewer days with ozone and PM2.5 (particles smaller than 2.5 microns) pollution levels exceeding the guidelines.[68]

In the UK, according to Roy Harrison, professor of environmental health at the University of Birmingham, it's "significantly healthier" to live in the countryside. Research shows that air pollution is responsible for an average loss of life expectancy of six months across the UK. Most of that is driven by urban populations.[69]

According to a study comparing air quality in cities, towns, and villages in central Poland, the level of air pollution depended largely on the size of the settlement unit. It was generally higher in the analyzed cities.[70]

In other words, according to available data, moving to the countryside is one possible solution if you value fresh air over the convenience of living in a city. If you're entertaining this idea, keep in mind there are caveats. Those living in less urban areas might not be exposed to the same high levels of ozone or PM2.5 pollution common in cities. But other sources of pollution can still affect the rural air quality. Air pollution can be a problem even for countryside residents. It's particularly prevalent in farming areas. That's where burning of crop residue, large scale use of tractor harvesters, pesticide and insecticide spraying, as well as grain dust can pose a risk to locals. This includes harm to those not involved with the daily farming tasks.

It pays to investigate the area where you want to move or where you spend your weekends. Less urban regions might not struggle with man-made air pollution, but they can still suffer from natural sources of pollution. For example, residents of little urbanized Big Island in Hawaii—a place where you'd think you'd enjoy excellent air quality as you sip a tropical cocktail while lying in a hammock—suffer from "vog," short for volcanic smog. It has become a part of everyday life for those living in areas downwind of the volcano Kīlauea.

One of the world's most active volcanoes, Mount Etna in Sicily, regularly spews lava and ash into the air. This causes poor air quality not only in the region around the volcano where many villages are, but even in the neighboring countries. It doesn't discern between city dwellers or suburban and rural residents.

Other natural pollutants that might be more common for those living in rural areas include wildfires. It's a problem known firsthand by those who live in the western United States and Canada. The dominant component of wildfire smoke, carbon dioxide, poses a low health risk via short-term exposure. However, the smoke also contains carbon monoxide, fine particulate matter, formaldehyde, acrolein, polyaromatic hydrocarbons, and benzene. These all pose a major threat. In the most extreme examples, wildfires lead not only to temporarily worse air quality, but to loss of life and property. This is what happened during the most destructive wildfire in California history in 2018. The bushfires of 2019 and 2020 in south-east Australia provide another sad example.

Dust storms that occur in the arid and semi-arid regions are another danger that affect air quality. This is regardless of whether you live in the city or in a less urban area. Residents of Arizona, New Mexico, eastern California, and west Texas are familiar with haboobs, intense dust storms occurring regularly in the dry regions.

In Europe, one notable example is Saharan Air Layer—winds blowing dust from a Saharan storm out over the Atlantic Ocean. Spanish Canary Islands, including the archipelago's two easternmost sparsely populated islands of Lanzarote and Fuerteventura, are regularly exposed to the phenomenon. They call it "calima" there. It's a hot, dry fog that irritates the airways, reduces visibility, and deposits a layer of fine dust over everything.

I asked a friend from the Canary Islands about her experience with calima. She joked that local meteorological agencies could hire her as a warning system. As an allergic, she can detect the dust coming before everyone else. Each time the Saharan sand blankets the islands, she suffers from dry eyes and respiratory problems. During one of the most extreme calimas, the visibility was so bad she couldn't see a building on the other side of the road. Soon, she, along with many other residents, landed in ER in desperate need of oxygen therapy. Calima might be a natural phenomenon, but it sure ain't fun, and it's unlikely you want to connect with this type of nature.

So, will moving to the countryside give you access to fresh air? The answer depends on where you want to move. Moving from the city to the countryside near a large farm can mean replacing one type of air pollution exposure to another. As Michigan State University toxicologist Jack Harkema notes, "In agricultural settings, you see some of the highest airborne concentrations of particulate matter due to dusty conditions generated by common agricultural practices." Studying the impact of air pollution on rural populations, Harkema emphasizes that "A lot of people think air pollution is just an urban issue, but we now know that it causes real problems in rural settings, too."[71]

If poor air quality in your city is a big problem and you want to move elsewhere, choosing the right environment is key to making sure that you get better access to fresh air. But if you're unwilling or unable to move, what can you do—if anything—to deal with this problem?

CHAPTER 7

Solutions: Combatting Air Pollution

૨૦

In chapter 5, where we talked about spending more time outside, there were many actions we could take to fix the issue. The big problem with air pollution is that on an individual scale there's little a single person can do to improve air quality. And yet, access to fresh air is not only important for our physical health. It's also key to our mental health as a species. We didn't evolve in a world so polluted that on some days we should even avoid going outside.

Of course, little decisions do matter. If everyone assumes that an individual can't do much to reduce air pollution, then no change will ever happen. Each of us has a tiny impact on air quality through our everyday choices. For example, using more environmentally friendly means of transportation does affect the level of pollution in your city and in your neighborhood. Using environmentally friendly sources of energy, including geothermal heating systems and solar panels helps. So does reducing or eliminating the use of the fireplace and wood stoves. So can help conserving energy and using energy-efficient appliances. Getting an energy audit done and making recommended improvements is another valuable undertaking. All energy that we consume needs to come from somewhere. That's often a local power plant producing toxic gases and particulate matter that we later breathe.

To improve air quality in the nearest vicinity of your home, consider planting a garden in your backyard. If you don't have one, potted plants on your balcony might also work on a small scale. As for choosing specific plants, the more leaves, the better. Leafy evergreen hedges, such as common ivy, are particularly effective at filtering air due to the extensive surface of their leaves.[72] Planting trees in your backyard, or on a larger scale, in your neighborhood, can provide a great benefit to the environment, too. They help trap a variety of pollutants, including ozone and nitrogen oxides as well as particulate matter.[73] Trees around the house increase its market value. If you live in a warm climate, extra shade has never hurt anyone. If you live in a cold climate, deciduous trees provide the best of both words: shade in the summer and light in the winter.

Everyone, both businesses and individuals, should take responsibility for the problem of air pollution. But before this change takes place on a grand scale, we need to do the next best thing we humans excel at: adapt. This starts with developing awareness of air pollution levels in your city. There are various sites where you can check them. My favorite site is https://aqicn.org with its real-time air pollution map for more than 100 countries. If air quality is poor, reconsider your plans for spending time outdoors, particularly if you want to exercise. During physical activity we breathe more deeply, often through the mouth. Consequently, the air bypasses nasal passages that normally filter airborne pollution particles.[74] Note that airing out your house during a period with low air quality doesn't make sense. I have a friend who can't open her windows on most winter days. The neighborhood is so polluted through the use of old coal-burning furnaces that her apartment would be instantly filled with smoke.

If you live in an area with high air pollution and opening windows isn't an option, consider investing in an indoor air purifier. If your house faces a busy street, let in fresh air through the rear windows. Conversely, if air quality is good, take advantage of the favorable conditions. Get your dose of natural light and fresh(er) air. Ventilate your house. Exercise outside. Breathe deeply.

Another way to deal with a city's air pollution is to avoid highly polluted areas. A team from King's College London analyzed seven popular routes through the city. They measured pollution exposure along main roads and backstreet routes. They found out that on average, taking the side street routes resulted in a 53 percent reduction in exposure to diesel fumes.[75] Diesel engines aren't common in the U.S. when compared to Europe. However, the general findings that there's lower air quality by the main roads hold true regardless of the type of fuel used. A review of more than 700 studies from around the world published by Health Effects Institute shows that the band within 0.2 to 0.3 miles (300 to 500 meters) of a highway is the area most highly affected by traffic emissions.[76] To avoid the worst of the air pollution, never exercise in the close vicinity of busy roads. Whenever possible, avoid walking by them altogether. If you do find yourself there, urban pollution consultant and researcher Dr. Iarla Kilbane-Dawe says that even walking further from the curb on a busy road has been shown to make a difference in pollution exposure.[77]

If you live in a city that struggles with extreme levels of pollution, wearing an anti-pollution mask might be sensible. This is most important if you spend extensive time in highly polluted areas, for example, when biking to work through heavy traffic. The most common and affordable anti-pollution masks are foldable 3M N95 masks. They filter out at least 95 percent of airborne particles larger than 0.3 microns. They need to fit well to offer maximum protection, though, which is often difficult to achieve.

Spend leisure time outside of the highly polluted urban areas. For your day trips, weekend trips, or vacations, choose destinations where you can breathe fresh air. As a nature lover, you don't need much encouragement to do it, do you? Even little everyday decisions about where you eat or where you exercise can lower your exposure. Jogging by a busy road will be more harmful to your health than heading out for a jog in a park. So will eating in a restaurant by a highway compared to eating in a restaurant in a low-traffic residential area. In the end, it all comes down to awareness and more deliberate choices as to where you decide to spend time, and thus, breathe the local air.

Protect yourself from the inside, too. Eat an antioxidant-rich, anti-inflammatory diet. According to experimental research at NYU School of Medicine, a plant-based diet such as the Mediterranean diet may protect people from the negative cardiopulmonary health effects of air pollution.[78] One of the study authors, Chris Lim, says that "Air pollution is hypothesized to cause bad health effects through oxidative stress and inflammation, and the Mediterranean diet is really rich in foods that are anti-inflammatory and have antioxidants that might intervene through those avenues."[79] According to Lim, it's the fruits, vegetables, and healthy fats that provide the protective benefits. A plant-rich diet is the healthiest diet anyway. You won't lose anything by increasing your intake of whole foods to protect yourself against the effects of breathing air of poor quality.

Here are the key actions to take to protect yourself against air pollution:

- Take responsibility for your own impact on local air quality. Conserve energy and keep the environment in mind as you go about your day.

- Surround yourself with plants, whether it be in your backyard or on your balcony, to trap a variety of pollutants.

- Develop awareness of air quality in your city. Spend more time outside when the air is fresh and protect yourself when it's not.

- Stay clear of highly polluted areas of your city. Whenever possible, avoid walking around main roads. If necessary, walk further from the curb to reduce your exposure to traffic emissions.

- When planning a day trip, a weekend trip, or your vacations, choose destinations that offer healthy air quality. Pay attention to fresh air also regarding where you spend your leisure time. Eating in a restaurant in a quiet neighborhood is better than in one right by a highway.

- Eat an antioxidant-rich, anti-inflammatory diet such as the Mediterranean diet to protect your body from the negative health effects of air pollution.

CHAPTER 8

Noise, Noise, Noise

ક

For more than a decade, bioacoustical scientist Kurt Fristrup and a small team of engineers, physicists, and biologists have been hiding microphones in parks and urban locations around the United States. Their goal? Measure noise levels in various environments. In each location, microphones measured decibel levels 33 times per second, 24 hours a day, for a month. The findings of the team were alarming, to say the least.

The urban locations are blaring. For example, Manhattan can be around 8,000 times louder than one of the quietest places in the contiguous U.S., Great Sand Dunes National Park and Preserve in south-central Colorado. Fristrup says that "There are times when I've been in the field in the intermountain west, where I've not only been able to hear my own heartbeat, but I've been able to hear the heartbeat of the person in the field with me."[80] In our urbanized areas, we're often lucky if we don't have to raise our voices to have a normal conversation while walking down the street.

The truth may be that noise pollution is the most pervasive ignored pollutant of our modern era. The noises that we make are astoundingly loud compared to natural sounds. The sound of leaves rustling is about 30 dBA (A-weighted decibels, used to measure environmental noise).[81] The sound of rainfall is about 50 dBA.[82] Meanwhile, the sound of heavy traffic is 85 dBA. The sound at a subway station is between 90 and 115 dBA. The sound of a motorcycle is between 95 and 110 dBA.[83]

A three dBA increase doubles the amount of noise (such an increase is barely noticeable to the human ear). A ten dBA increase makes noise ten times louder. A 20 dBA increase makes it 100 times louder. This means that a noisy restaurant at 80 dBA is 100 times louder than a normal conversation at 60 dBA.

One of the loudest noises nature makes, the sound of a thunder (let's ignore ear-splitting volcanic eruptions) is 120 dBA. This is as loud as a band concert. But it's still not as loud as countless man-made noises, including a chain saw at 125 dBA or a power drill at 130 dBA. I haven't even mentioned an airplane taking off at 140 dBA, or a shotgun at 170 dBA.

A lion or tiger can roar as loud as 114 decibels, which is about 25 times louder than a gas-powered lawn mower[84] but still much quieter than a chain saw. Only the loudest recorded bird call (the white bellbird) can match the chain saw noise at 125 decibels.[85] And we're talking about the loudest bird. An average bird's song will be drowned out by the sounds of traffic.

Loud natural sounds, unlike so many urban sounds, are *occasional.* You don't hear them all the time when you're on a hike in the wilderness. Before our modern civilization began, our ancestors were never continuously exposed to noise that would damage their health. They didn't live by busy streets and airports. Neither they lived in a neighborhood where everyone seemed to be mowing the lawn at the same exact time, using a lawnmower that sounds like it was designed to show off how loud it is (no, I'm not a fan of lawnmowers).

Excess noise can have drastic consequences on our health. Delhi is one of the noisiest cities in the world. According to the Worldwide Hearing Index 2017 created by Mimi Hearing Technologies, the residents of this city on average suffer a hearing loss equal to someone 19 years older than them.[86] But it's one of the noisiest cities in the world so if you don't live there, you're safe, right? Here's the kicker. Even in Vienna, the city that scored best in the ranking, the study participants had a hearing loss equal to someone more than 10 years older than them.

You can test your own hearing with the company's smartphone app Mimi Hearing Test. The app plays background noise and asks you to hold the button when you hear the beep. I'm happy to report that my test showed that my hearing grade is excellent.

According to the results of the Worldwide Hearing Index 2017 study, there was a 64 percent correlation between hearing loss and noise pollution. This indicates that hearing loss may be an outcome of or be partly caused by living in the studied cities. But, of course, correlation doesn't imply causation. This is even when it's obvious that city dwellers are exposed to more noise pollution than rural residents. The findings show that the countries with the highest overall combined hearing loss include: India, United Arab Emirates, Turkey, Israel, Brazil, and Ukraine. The countries that suffer the least include: Canada, Japan, Romania, Austria, Switzerland, Germany, and Sweden.

Wild nature is not silent. Animals make sounds when they communicate with each other. Waves crash on the beach. Rocks fall with a loud bang. Wind can be howling. Rain can be pelting. Thunders can be deafening. But the baseline level of noise in a natural setting is non-existent compared to the built environment. Also, unlike urban sounds, most natural sounds don't provoke annoyance. There are exceptions, but as a whole, it's the man-made noises that drive us insane. I can listen to bird songs all day long. The noise generated by an aerobatic plane flying over my house (living close to a small airport doesn't help) makes me go postal.

Excess noise may cause cardiovascular conditions and affect cognition in the elderly.[87] It was associated with an increased incidence of: arterial hypertension, myocardial infarction, heart failure, and stroke.[88] And of course, there's also a risk of noise-induced hearing loss,[89] which the results of the Worldwide Hearing Index 2017 make rather clear.

So how often are we exposed to noise that can affect our health on such a deep level? Unfortunately, more often than we think. The recommended maximum 24-hour average noise exposure is 55 dBA. Exposures above this level may increase the risk of hypertension.[90] Sadly, in the U.S., about 45 percent of the population is exposed to annual levels over 55 dBA. In Europe, it's 23 percent of the population (data for 33 European Environment Agency countries).[91] Moving on to even louder noise and even worse consequences, according to The National Institute for Occupational Safety and Health in the U.S., exposures at or above 85 dBA cause possible damage in just eight hours.[92] This isn't the level of noise generated by power tools. It's merely as loud as the noise of heavy traffic or the noise inside a busy restaurant.[93]

How about wilderness in the modern world?

Acoustic ecologist Gordon Hempton is on a mission to preserve silence in the wilderness. He lives near the Olympic National Park in the rugged northwest corner of Washington State. According to his research, that's where you can find the quietest place in the contiguous United States. More specifically, the least noise polluted place is in the Hoh Rain Forest. The quietest spot is approximately three miles from the visitors center. The ecologist placed a small red stone to mark this special place. You can listen to a free preview and buy an unedited 72-minute recording from this area from Hempton's website at www.soundtracker.com.)

Audio technician Mike Mikkelsen, working for Hempton's foundation One Square Inch of Silence, explains, "In a place like this your auditory horizon isn't just 1 or 2 miles. You can hear everything that's happening in this valley. … It's like we're listening to 5 miles or 10 miles around us right now."[94]

The red stone marks one of fewer than ten naturally quiet places in the lower 48, defined by Hempton as a place where each day there's at least a 15-minute period free of man-made sounds. That's not a typo: *fifteen* minutes without man-made sounds. When I first learned how few such places were left, I was shocked. Noise is so prevalent in our modern lives that we can't escape it even in the wilderness.

Unfortunately, besides the places identified by Hempton, there's nowhere in the contiguous U.S. where it's possible to find more than a brief respite from man-made noises. In Europe, according to his estimates, there are no such places left. In most of the national parks in the U.S., the daytime, noise-free interval is five minutes or less.[95] The cause: airplanes. Many of us are so used to them that we don't hear them unless we focus. But the sounds are there, day in, day out, affecting wildlife[96] and possibly our recovery after psychological stress.[97] German scientists have also established a potential link between aircraft noise and depression and anxiety. The prevalence of these disorders increased twofold in the presence of strong noise annoyance.[98]

We don't need scientific research to prove that rural areas are better if you want to escape the most annoying, pervasive urban sounds. Car horns, incessant jackhammering sounds from construction sites, various machines and appliances, and loud music are less prevalent in the countryside. It's not complete silence, though. As Hempton's research shows, you can't escape man-made noise even in some of the wildest places in the lower 48. But you can still hear the difference between an urbanized and a rural area loud and clear.

When you look at the sound map provided by the National Park Service,[99] you'll notice that the less urbanized states have lower levels of noise compared to highly urbanized areas. For example, the least urbanized state in the U.S., Maine, is mostly blue (indicating low noise) on the map. Meanwhile, the area extending from Washington, D.C. to New York City (as well as any other major city) is lit up yellow. This indicates high levels of noise. A sound map provided by the European Environment Agency shows similar findings. Those who live in urban areas are most affected by road traffic, which is the main source of environmental noise in Europe.[100]

Even if rural areas may save our hearing and sanity, not all of us want to leave our urban lives behind. Can urbanites find any peace in a city, or is noise unescapable?

CHAPTER 9

Solutions: Combatting Noise Pollution

❧

Living in a city, it's impossible to enjoy the silence our ancestors took for granted. But it doesn't mean there's nothing we can do to protect our ears and our sanity.

Dealing with noise pollution starts with developing awareness of how much noise surrounds you. You then reclaim control of the problem instead of assuming you can't fix it because you live in a city. Your everyday choices make a significant impact on your noise exposure. Do you often go to busy, crowded restaurants or cook at home in a quieter environment? Do you exercise at a gym that plays loud music or use headphones for an even more direct assault on your ears? Do you go shopping during the busy hours or choose to go when there are few people around? Do you often go to concerts, sports games, and other events with hazardous noise levels or prefer quieter activities?

As a guest, customer, or patron, do you voice your opinion when a venue plays music too loud? Restaurants are particularly guilty of this. On more than several occasions I was forced to ask for the music to be turned down or to request a table in a quieter spot. This is not being difficult. If you're polite, you have the right to voice your displeasure as a paying customer.

How often do you seek tranquil spaces in nature or at the least a quiet environment like a library? Bombarding ourselves with hustle and bustle carries consequences not only for our hearing. It also has an impact on our mental and physical health. We've evolved in a world that was, for the most part, quiet and low-stimuli. Wouldn't it make sense to try to recreate at least a shadow of this world, particularly in our living spaces?

Consider the background noises in your house: the fridge, dishwasher, washing machine, vacuum cleaner, or your lawn mower. What if instead of complaining about the noise, you replaced old, noisy appliances with new, quieter models?

I once lived in a small apartment with an old fridge that produced loud, gargling sounds every fifteen minutes. As you can imagine, getting quality sleep was a challenge. I lasted two weeks before I had to move (the place being a cheap apartment, the landlord wouldn't replace it). When I was shopping for my first fridge, can you guess what feature it needed to have? You guessed right: I wanted the quietest model available on the market.

What other sources of noise bother you in your house, and how can you reduce them? Even small changes, when combined, can result in big improvements. You could have carried a comfortable whispering conversation in a cave where our ancestors lived. Can you do the same in your own house? We might never reach or even desire the same level of tranquility in our modern homes. Lowering the noise level can still make us healthier, though.

Let's move on to external noises we can't control that easily. If you live by a busy road or other source of noise, closing the windows might be the only effective solution. This goes against what we discussed about indoor pollution. It doesn't mean you have to keep your windows closed all the time, though. Air out your room in the early morning or before you go to sleep. Keep the windows closed during the day when the noise is most annoying. Consider soundproofing your house. If you have old leaky windows, replace them with ones that are more effective at blocking noise. At the expense of blocking daylight from coming inside, you can also install noise-reducing curtains. A more budget-friendly natural solution is a windowsill garden that may also help reduce noise coming in from the cracks in the windows. Even a rolled blanket (perhaps with a natural pattern) can help lower indoor noise levels. Improving insulation—materials used on the walls, ceilings, and floors—can also help absorb noise.

When I replaced windows in my apartment, the level of noise dropped dramatically. In hindsight, it was obvious this would happen. The old windows were so damaged you could feel air entering through the cracks. Yet the difference was still striking. It's an expensive investment, but shouldn't home be a quiet place to recharge? If you can't reduce the noise originating from outside your home, you can make it more bearable by using a white noise machine. You can also put on a playlist with natural sounds like waves crashing on the beach, rainfall, or water flowing down a stream. Dense shrubs and hedges planted around your house can also reduce noise levels. If you can't plant anything around your house, you can consider installing bamboo or wicker screens (bonus points for using a natural, renewable material).

I love summer, but each year I also dread what's coming along with it: neighbors working on their remodeling projects. As a person living in an apartment in a multi-family building, there's always someone starting a renovation project. What follows is incessant noise ruining any chances of enjoying a quiet afternoon on the balcony. If you're sensitive to noise and live in a similar neighborhood, moving to a single-family detached home might be the only remedy (yours truly is so tired of noise that he does have a plan to move, too).

Protecting yourself as you go about your business in the city is also important. Again, our ancestors never spent countless hours in loud environments with irritating, hearing-damaging sounds surrounding them all the time. Using noise-canceling headphones or earplugs might not be the most practical solution at the office. They can be a godsend, however, when commuting in a loud metro, on a flight, or when using loud appliances and power tools. Don't discount the importance of work hygiene. It's not "just" harmless thirty minutes mowing the lawn without protection. Not wearing proper protection when using loud tools can lead to lasting, unenjoyable consequences.

On a lifestyle note, allow yourself to enjoy some silence during your leisure time. How often do you let yourself enjoy silence at home without listening to anything? Is there always something on in the background—music, a podcast, an audiobook? Turn it off at least every now and then—constant (man-made) noise isn't natural for us. Reconnect with your roots daily through a peaceful, quiet repose, even if it's for two minutes.

Whether you're exploring the wilderness, having a picnic at the beach, or jogging in a local urban park, keep your voice down, too. Avoid shouting, and if you must listen to music, use earbuds over external speakers. Making unnecessary noise in public areas, particularly in nature, is equal to littering. Would you go about your local park and trash it? If not, please don't spoil it with noise pollution, either. Following these simple rules makes life easier and more enjoyable for all of us.

Here are the key actions to take to combat noise pollution:

- Develop awareness about how much noise surrounds you. Become more conscious of how and where you spend time. Aim to spend less time in noisy environments and more in tranquil ones. Protect your hearing in loud venues such as in a metro or on a flight or when working with loud machines.

- Take stock of background noises in your house. Reduce them through replacing old appliances.

- Pay attention to external noises and devise strategies to soundproof your house. You can accomplish that through replacing old leaky windows. Installing noise-reducing curtains is another option. Something as simple as rolled blankets on a windowsill can also help. For a bonus dose of nature, some potted plants can also help block some noise.

- If you can't reduce outside noises, drown them out by using a white noise machine or listening to natural sounds.

- To reduce noise generated by street traffic, consider planting dense shrubs around your property. If not possible, install bamboo or wicker screens.

❧ Let yourself enjoy some silence at home. Even if for just a few minutes, turn off music, radio, a podcast or an audiobook and enjoy the quietude.

❧ Be considerate when spending time in public areas, particularly in a natural setting. Making unnecessary noises is like littering.

CHAPTER 10

The Worrisome Case of
the Missing Stars

 za

It was 4:30 in the morning on January 17, 1994, when a 6.7-magnitude earthquake woke up the residents of Los Angeles. A massive blackout followed, thrusting the city into darkness. Those who left their houses to check on the neighborhood were so shocked when they looked at the sky that they called 911. They reported a "giant silvery cloud" over the city. Apparently, it looked so sinister that they thought the world was ending.

But it was just the good old Milky Way. It was the very same one that every human around the world once saw in its entire glory every cloudless night. It's the same one which now, thanks to the 24/7 artificial light, some people have never seen in their lives.[101]

It's ironic that we don't get sufficient natural light exposure during the day, but we get excess artificial light at night (ALAN). According to a meta-analysis of the effects of ALAN on human health, it leads to:

- circadian rhythm disruptions,
- sleep disorders,
- breast cancer (artificial light at night disrupts sleep-promoting hormone melatonin production, which then affects the release of estrogen),
- a possible negative impact on psychological, cardiovascular, and metabolic functions.[102]

The sad truth is that 80 percent of the world and more than 99 percent of the U.S. and European populations live under light-polluted skies, detached from one of the most beautiful natural sights. Overall, the Milky Way is hidden from more than one-third of humanity. This includes 60 percent of Europeans and nearly 80 percent of North Americans.[103] The loss of visibility not only impacts health, but also represents the loss of a powerful symbol. Instead of watching the sky lit up by stars, we're left with the dull, orange skyglow of the city. How are children supposed to reach for the stars if they can't even see them?

The scale of the problem is underreported and ignored, but it doesn't mean it's without consequence. The most light-polluted country in the world, Singapore, is so brightly lit that the entire population lives under skies so bright the eye can't fully adapt to night vision.[104] The city is applauded for its many nature-friendly initiatives, but caring for starry nights is not one of them. Abundant artificial lighting makes the sky so bright at night you can't see the stars unless you leave the country. The eyes of the residents never get to experience true natural darkness.

Light pollution is also harmful for the natural environment. The energy costs are immense, straining already overexploited resources. Then there's the large impact on fauna and flora. According to ecologist Franz Hölker of Germany's Leibniz-Institute for Freshwater Ecology and Inland Fisheries, light pollution has consequences for 30 percent of nocturnal vertebrates. It also impacts more than 60 percent of nocturnal invertebrates. The affected animals change their natural night habits such as reproduction and migration. The problem also affects plants and microorganisms.[105]

City-dwelling nature lovers can't do much to be able to see the Milky Way. To make matters worse, if they want to get away to enjoy starry nights, they need to be at a large distance from the nearest city to avoid light pollution. Los Angeles is so brightly lit that you can see its nighttime lights, resembling a sunrise, from a rural road 90 miles away (145 kilometers).[106] The lights of Las Vegas are visible as a glow on the horizon from 90 miles away, too.

Does this mean that light pollution is a sad fact of life for those who are unwilling to live in the countryside away from urban areas? Thankfully, there's some hope: International Dark Sky Communities. They are places certified by International Dark-Sky Association that have shown "exceptional dedication to the preservation of the night sky through the implementation and enforcement of a quality outdoor lighting ordinance, dark sky education and citizen support of dark skies."[107]

In the U.S., some of the most populated International Dark Sky Communities include Flagstaff, Fountain Hills, Cottonwood, Camp Verde, and Sedona in Arizona; Dripping Springs, Horseshoe Bay, and Wimberley in Texas; Homer Glen in Illinois; and Ketchum in Idaho.

In Canada, the small town of Bon Accord in central Alberta enjoys this designation. In Europe, apart from three small, sparsely populated islands in Scotland, Denmark, and Guernsey, only two International Dark Sky Communities could be called urban areas: Fulda in Germany and Moffat in Scotland.

One can hope that thanks to these examples, more cities and towns will adapt practices that will help their citizens enjoy starry nights.

International Dark-Sky Association also designates International Dark Sky Parks. It's "a land possessing an exceptional or distinguished quality of starry nights and a nocturnal environment that is specifically protected for its scientific, natural, educational, cultural heritage, and/or public enjoyment."[108] Living close to one of the Dark Sky Parks could be another alternative to gain access to what our ancestors took for granted. In the U.S., Arizona is home to more certified Dark Sky Places than anywhere else in the world. Internationally, such parks also exist in: Australia, Croatia, Denmark, Germany, Hungary, Ireland, Israel, Japan, Netherlands, South Korea, Spain, and the United Kingdom.

The negative health effects of light also apply on a smaller scale. We've grown accustomed to using electronic devices throughout the day. This includes using them in the evening and at night when our eyes aren't supposed to be exposed to light. Research shows that the use of these devices before bedtime increases the time it takes to fall asleep. It also disrupts the circadian clock, suppresses levels of melatonin, and reduces the amount and delays the timing of restorative REM sleep. As a consequence, the use of electronic devices at night reduces alertness the following morning.[109] After sunset, our ancestors could only rely on fire, which cast a weak, warm light. It was like no light at all compared to our modern lightbulbs and devices that trick our bodies into thinking the day hasn't yet ended. Combined with light pollution outside, it's no wonder that so many of us suffer from sleep disorders and struggle to rest at night.

Light pollution isn't as common a topic as air pollution. It doesn't mean we can ignore this harmful, unnatural aspect of living in a city, though. What's above our heads on a starry night is as important a part of nature as the oceans, forests, and mountains around us. So, what if we don't plan to move to an unlit rural area or a Dark Sky Community or Park? What can we do to deal with this problem?

CHAPTER 11

Solutions: Minimizing Light Pollution

২৯

A s with air pollution, there's unfortunately little an average city dweller can do to reduce light pollution levels in their city. The only action you can take that might improve the local area is to optimize outdoor lighting by your house. Perhaps there's no need for lighting or the lights don't have to be that strong. Consider using motion sensors instead of leaving the lights on for the entire night. Lights placed lower, ideally shielded pathway bollards that illuminate the ground instead of the sky, also reduce the amount of pollution. Using lights with lower color temperatures (warm lights) helps reduce exposure to blue light at night. International Dark-Sky Association recommends using outdoor lighting that has a color temperature of no more than 3,000 Kelvins.[110]

With your own backyard taken care of, act when unwanted light enters your property. Your neighbor might not even know when a bright light from their property shines over the fence into your backyard, or worse, inside your home. If streetlights bother you, reach out to a local government agency responsible for maintaining them. Ask to shield the lights or take other measures to change the direction of the light. Streetlights, as the name implies, should only illuminate the street below them, not houses in their vicinity.

If you can't eliminate the external sources of light, limit your exposure with physical barriers. The same shades, curtains, drapes, and blinds whose use you should limit during the day can be useful at night. This is key if you live in an area with brightly lit buildings or surrounded by strong artificial lights coming from billboards, passing cars, etc.

To further protect yourself from the effects of artificial light at night, turn off unnecessary lights. Reduce the use of electronic devices, too. This includes smartphones, tablets, laptops, or e-readers with built-in light. As we've explored in the previous chapter, the use of these devices carries significant negative consequences.

Most of us use electronic devices before going to sleep (yours truly included). Let's keep it real—it's unlikely we'll stop using them altogether in the evening. Our ancestors might have survived without those conveniences. We, however, are too addicted to them at this point to forgo them completely. But even a small change can help. For example, don't use them within 15 to 30 minutes of going to sleep. Read on an e-reader without built-in light. Opt for a paper book or an audiobook. You can also change the color temperature of certain devices to reduce the amount of sleep-disrupting blue light they emit. In your smartphone, it's called a "night shift" or a "night light" setting. From the perspective of our sleep quality, the less light at night, the better. It's a primary signal for the body to start winding down. By making our homes resemble the pitch-black caves inhabited by our ancestors, we can get better quality sleep and perform better during the day, too.

Here are the key actions to take to reduce the negative impact of light pollution on our lives:

- Optimize outdoor lighting by your house. Turn off unnecessary lights. Use lighting of a color temperature of no more than 3,000 Kelvins. Aim to illuminate only the specific area you want to keep bright, such as a pathway, instead of the sky.

- Act when unwanted light enters your property to educate others on the dangers of light pollution.

- If you can't eliminate the external sources of light, protect yourself by using shades, curtains, drapes, and blinds.

🕭 Reduce the use of electronic devices before going to bed. As light pollution outside, this habit will impact your sleep and well-being. Replace e-readers and tablets with paper books or audiobooks. Use night light mode on your smartphone.

CHAPTER 12

The Shrinking Space in Our Growing Cities

ટ

I was close to snapping. The crowds in the supermarket were so large that I repeatedly bumped into people and people bumped into me. The atmosphere was tense. Nobody enjoys their shopping to resemble a sold-out concert. Then there was an endless wait in a line. Then I couldn't leave the parking lot as a mini traffic jam formed. Then a careless driver almost crashed into me as I was exiting the premises. I was stressed out and angry for the rest of the morning. In hindsight, it wasn't a big deal. Nothing horrible happened. It was just a busy day in a supermarket. Yet, the situation shows how stressful living in a city with dense population can be.

Humans need sufficient space to feel good. Confined to small apartments in congested cities, many urbanites don't get to enjoy wide, open spaces. Rarely can they experience much needed solitude or breathe more deeply without feeling boxed in. And it's yet another example of urban life clashing with our inner wiring.

For most of our history, we lived in small tribes. On any given day, we might have interacted with a few dozen individuals, all of whom we knew. Today, we don't even know our neighbors, let alone even a percentile of people living in our city. The feeling of community is gone for many residents of big cities as well as many towns. There's a reason for that: living in such a huge cluster is not in our inner wiring.

British anthropologist Robin Dunbar puts the number of a cohesive network of meaningful contacts at 150. Go above 150, and a group splits off or collapses. The same theory suggests that we can recognize at most 1,500 people.[111] And here we are living in cities with millions of residents where you can see 1,500 strangers any given minute. To make matters worse, because of high population density, those people often intrude on our personal space. Crowding, or being crowded, as my supermarket experience shows, is yet another inconvenience of urban living that impacts our well-being.

The feeling of being crowded is a relatively new development in human history. According to Colin Ellard, a professor of cognitive neuroscience at Canada's University of Waterloo, "Living in a city is an unnatural state for human beings. [We evolved] living in small groups of around 100 to 150 people." Ellard studies the impact of places on the brain and body. He explains the impact of crowded places on our health in the following manner:

> There are two ways in which [living] in large cities exerts a psychological toll: one is the physical stress of crowding, which includes noise, but also the feeling of being crowded at high density with other people. This alone is known to cause powerful stress responses—commuters on packed buses have higher levels of cortisol, a hormone associated with stress. The second psychological liability of city life comes from being in constant contact with strangers. This state of affairs can lead to feelings of social isolation and loneliness, and then of course have mental health consequences.[112]

There's an entire field of study called proxemics dedicated to the human use of space and the effects that population density has on our behaviors, communication, and social interaction. Cultural anthropologist Edward T. Hall coined the term in 1963. In his book *The Hidden Dimension*, he explained four interpersonal distances. The first one is intimate space, for embracing, hugging and whispering. The second one is personal space for interactions with friends and family. The third one is social space for interactions among acquaintances. The final one is public space for public speaking.

And here's the big problem of urban living that clashes with our inner wiring. Strangers notoriously intrude on the spaces reserved for our lovers, families, or friends. It doesn't feel good. We experience discomfort, anger, or anxiety when someone uninvited encroaches on our personal zone. We feel awkward, if not outright attacked, when that old lady breathes right into our ear in a supermarket line and can't get a hint that she's standing too close. Rubbing against other people in a crowded bus or train doesn't feel good, either. In fact, our brains do indeed consider unwanted presence in our personal space as a *threat*. The process is regulated by the amygdala, a part of the brain responsible for processing, among others, emotional responses.[113] In the past, strangers getting too close to us was how problems started. Today, it's how we live.

Invading the personal space of animals usually leads to one of two instinctual reactions: fight or flight. In our modern civilization, barring extreme circumstances, we don't employ the former, so we opt for the latter. Only we can't escape. The usual measures like stepping back, taking as little space as possible, or avoiding eye contact might help reduce some discomfort, but they don't eliminate it. Our fight-or-flight response, designed to deal with occasional, extreme situations, kicks in repeatedly each day. It's no wonder we're so stressed out and exhausted after a long commute or merely spending a lot of time in a densely populated area. We humans like our space. But space is a precious, limited resource in a city.

A study on preferred interpersonal distances around the world shows that the amount of personal space we need is influenced by one's culture and personal preferences.[114] In Romania, Hungary, Saudi Arabia, and Turkey, average social distance reserved for a stranger is more than four feet (120 cm), Meanwhile, in Ukraine, Bulgaria, Peru, and Argentina, this distance is less than three feet (90 cm). Americans and Brits need on average a little more than three feet of distance for strangers. Most countries fall somewhere between three to four feet.

How often do other city dwellers get well into our three to four feet of personal space? When using public transportation, all the time. When walking down a busy sidewalk, all the time. When standing anywhere in a line, all the time. We can't escape it. It's a fact of life that if you spend any time in a city, on any given day, people will bump into you and provoke a fight or flight reaction. Some of us fare better with crowds than others. Humans can adapt. An unwanted intrusion will be a minor nuisance for a person frequently exposed to crowds and a major frustration to someone who avoids them.

Our personal preferences may be also influenced by our childhood and our standards. A child growing up in a small village in the wide-open spaces of Greenland, a territory with the lowest population density in the world, will be used to having more personal space and more space to live in general. Their expectation is one of a lot of space. That's what the environment in which they grew up offered in spades. Meanwhile, a child in Macau, a territory with the highest population density in the world, won't be as bothered by crowds. Their personal space threshold will be smaller.

I grew up in a quiet neighborhood right by an urban forest. Even though it was a mid-sized city, I spent most of my time playing in nature, away from other people. With a couple of close friends, we used to spend most of our time in what we called "bases" (as in, "military bases"). They were our hideaways in thick, tall bushes or in small trees with spreading canopies. As an introvert, I hated going to kindergarten and later, school, where there were so many kids around and so little personal space. To this day, I don't feel comfortable around crowds. Whenever I visit a bigger city, I feel claustrophobic and trapped. A part of it might be influenced by my personality. Yet, there's no doubt that had I grown up in a different environment with less space and more people around, I would have a different tolerance level. Following this train of thought, if you spend considerable time out in nature, crowds might bother you more, too. In contrast, faithful urbanites who are surrounded by crowds daily might not share the same expectations.

Speaking of space, let's travel back in time to the Serengeti. Treeless grasslands, open woodlands, nothing in sight but wide, open spaces. Humans evolved with *a lot* of space around them. Even if they huddled in a cave at night, they had the entire natural world around them during the day. Their views weren't blocked by skyscrapers. Barring natural features like mountains, rivers, lakes, and oceans, they could go in any direction they wanted. Their vistas often extended as far as the eye could see. Today, city dwellers, particularly those residing in the largest cities with the highest population density, live in the equivalent of a prison to our free-roaming ancestors.

And what about the effects of personality on how we handle space? Well, introverts, who comprise an estimated 33 to 50 percent of the American population according to Susan Cain, bestselling author of *Quiet: The Power of Introverts in a World That Can't Stop Talking*, may suffer from lack of space even more than other city dwellers. That's because they need quiet, private places to recharge. If there are humans everywhere you go, it can be difficult as an introvert to meet your need for solitude. Unfortunately, urban parks and other public spaces are often full of people. This can further intensify the anxiety of being trapped. Hiding at home becomes the only option for introverts seeking some solitude. It's a conundrum because we've already discussed that spending too much time indoors doesn't serve us. But this problem isn't limited to introverts alone. Even a person who prefers to recharge through socializing sometimes needs some time alone. Whether you're a social butterfly or a loner, if you can't find a quiet space in your city when you need it, you may feel hemmed in by the concrete jungle around you.

This lack of space in cities has another potential health consequence: myopia. We've already learned that because children don't get enough natural light anymore, more of them have myopia. But there's also another potential reason the condition might be rising in urban areas. According to biomechanist and bestselling author Katy Bowman, we don't look over all the distances now, limiting ourselves to objects close to us.[115] In her book *Movement Matters: Essays on Movement Science, Movement Ecology, and the Nature of Movement*, she points out an interesting fact. Assuming that a human eye can focus on an object up to a mile (1.6 kilometers) away (studies put this theoretical number at closer to 1.6 miles or 2.6 kilometers),[116] city dwellers limit the use of their eyes to less than a half of a percent of their ocular range of focus.

We almost exclusively focus on activities done at short working distance such as reading, writing, studying, or using a smartphone. Even when we look beyond the screens, we don't look at distances longer than perhaps 20 feet away (six meters).

It's a plausible theory. When we don't use the full range of motion of our muscles, we eventually find ourselves unable to achieve certain natural positions (for example, a full squat). In the same way, if we don't use the full range of motion of our eyes, they might lose the ability to see over all the distances. So, the solution is simple: let's look through the window. Problem solved. If it were only so simple. To achieve the full range of motion of our eyes, we would first need to be able to have an unobstructed view for a mile (or 1.6 miles depending on the estimates). Unless you live in a penthouse in the tallest building in your city, it's unlikely you'll be able to see that far. Countless structures will block the horizon. Of course, you'll get some benefits of looking at far objects, but they won't be as far away as the eye could (and should) see.

From the windows in my apartment I can see at most about 1,000 feet (300 meters) away. That's not even 20 percent of Bowman's estimate and less than 10 percent of the distance estimated by researchers. Sneaking into a tall building each time I want to exercise my eyes would be impractical, so I need to leave the city to be able to see over long distances.

But this brings us to yet another problem. We could escape to the wilderness to find some peace and look at the faraway horizon. The sad reality of many popular national parks, though, is that they're overcrowded. One of the wildest areas in Poland are the Tatra Mountains in the south. Unfortunately, the most popular trails are so crowded that people often have to wait up to a few hours in a line to get to the peak, take a few pictures, and descend while bumping into others waiting their turn. It's hardly a restorative experience in quiet, natural surroundings.

In the U.S., many of the most popular national parks are forced to limit the number of visitors by requiring backcountry permits. For example, one of the most coveted permits, the permit to hike the John Muir Trail, is processed by lottery 24 weeks (168 days) in advance of the hiking start date.[117] Even the rugged Glacier National Park in Montana, distant from major cities, takes reservations. As the National Park Service suggests on their website, "Securing an advance reservation before you get to Glacier can eliminate the stress of competing for a walk-in permit at the height of the busy summer season."[118]

It's sad that we need to "compete" for a chance to enjoy those wild places. But it seems to be the only way to preserve them and ensure that those who do get the chance to visit them can have an uncrowded experience. With so many people craving connection with nature, finding peace, both in the city and in the wilderness, takes more effort. Thankfully, it's still achievable.

For example, on a trip to Bieszczady Mountains, one of the wildest and least populated areas in Poland, to avoid crowds resembling a busy downtown, my friends and I sought recently opened or little-known trails. If we had headed to the most popular trails, we would have been sharing the experience with thousands of people. It took a bit more work to enjoy a quiet, restorative hike, but it could be done. On a trip to Tenerife in the Canary Islands, my friend and I decided to start our descent down the Masca Gorge, a popular hiking route, before the first light. Thanks to our dedication, on our way down we met a handful of people. On our way back up we passed hundreds of people. Just two hours later the quiet early morning hike in the peaceful valley turned into the complete opposite of why we headed there in the first place. But at least we enjoyed it during our way down.

What if living in a crowded city and periodically going on wilderness trips doesn't satisfy your need for more space? Would moving to a rural or less urban area help? The answer is a resounding yes. This is of course not surprising, but what might be surprising is how big of a difference merely moving to a smaller town close to a major city can make.

For example, the population density in New York City is 27,751 per square mile (10,715 per square kilometer). Meanwhile, the town of Mount Pleasant, New York, less than an hour by car from NYC, has a population density of 1,623 per square mile (626 per square kilometer). That's 17 times lower than NYC. The town of Bedford, New York, close to Ward Pound Ridge Reservation, has a population density that's four times lower than Mount Pleasant. It's almost 58 times lower than NYC: 482 per square mile (186 per square kilometer). It's just an hour by car from one of the biggest cities in the world.

Those towns are still urbanized areas with all their conveniences, yet they offer breathing space the bustling city can't provide. If you're willing to move to a rural area, the number of people sharing each square mile drops dramatically. The village of Speculator, New York, located within the Adirondack Park, the largest park in the contiguous United States, has a population density of just seven people per square mile (3 per kilometer).

If you're craving space, you'll find it in rural areas in spades. But what are the solutions for those city dwellers who can't or don't want to move to less urban areas? How can you combat the loss of space as an urbanite?

CHAPTER 13

Solutions: Combatting the Loss of Space

ᚥ

If we had magic wands, the best solution would be to create magical bubbles around us to keep strangers from intruding on our personal space. But since such devices aren't invented (yet?), the best we can do is—yet again—develop more awareness of the problem and avoid crowded areas.

While it sounds obvious, how often do you go out of your way to give yourself a break from the crowds? If I told you it could reduce your stress levels, would you start paying more attention to your crowd exposure? Our personal spaces might be shrinking as we live in increasingly more-crowded cities. This doesn't mean it's natural for us or carries no consequences.

Of course, you might not be able to avoid people when using public transportation, but you can choose how you spend your free time. For example, you can go to your favorite restaurant during the less busy hours. Google where you want to go, and you'll see popular hours each day of the week. You can also order take-out and enjoy it at home in solitude. In the same way, you can adjust your schedule regarding when you go to the gym. If you need to go at all, that is—perhaps you can build a home gym or exercise in a natural, non-gym environment? Adjust your schedule for other public venues like a theater, supermarket (unless you stumble upon a random rush hour like I did), or even your local park, too. Your amygdala will thank you for that.

If possible, commuting by means of transportation other than a crowded metro or bus might be another potential solution. Commuting by car is best from the perspective of avoiding strangers invading your personal space. It carries undeniable environmental consequences, though. You're also replacing one type of stress (crowds) with another (traffic jams, which also, in a way, lead to a feeling of being crowded). Carpooling is one way of reducing costs and the environmental impact, although it's still not as efficient as public transportation. Biking or walking is a great option if you live close to the office. It also has a drawback, though. You might be exchanging one set of problems for another. You avoid crowds but increase your exposure to air pollution. Then there's also an increased risk of an accident if you live in a bike-unfriendly city.

Become your city's explorer and find quiet urban places with few people around. This might take a little work, but it can be done. You might not be able to find a place where you'll be all by yourself for hours on end. So, the goal is to find your personal sanctuary in the city that helps you relax for at least fifteen minutes. Even on short visits as a person not familiarized with the city, I have been able to find relatively quiet and uncrowded places all around the world. For example, I found them in Polish cities of Warsaw, Łódź and Gdańsk (population of 1.7 million, 720,000, and 575,000 respectively). It was also possible in Singapore with its 5.6 million residents. Given the country's pro-environmental tendencies, it's easy to find a quiet spot, though. Doha in Qatar, with almost 800,000 inhabitants, was also empty in certain areas. Extreme heat keeps people indoors in this part of the world. Phoenix, Arizona with 1.6 million people, also has its quiet spots. As a resident of your own city, you might already know which parts are the quietest and where you can escape the hustle and bustle.

To combat the myopia risk, exercise your eyes by regularly looking as far away as you can see, ideally in a natural setting. Looking through the window is better than nothing. But it's best to find a place where you have an unobstructed view for at least a mile (1.6 kilometers) and preferably 1.6 miles (2.6 kilometers). Bridges, skyscrapers, and other similar tall, man-made structures can help in this aspect, too. If you're blessed to live by the ocean or sea, you have a perfect place to look over long distances. If you need another reason to be on the beach as often as possible, add eye health benefits to your list.

If you're struggling to find a place where you can look over long distances, consider sky gazing. You can try to spot airplanes (pretty easy), birds (a bit harder), unusual cloud formations, stars, satellites, and other interesting objects in the sky. This is not the same as a panoramic view over the landscape around you but it's better than nothing.

As you seek wide open spaces outside of urban settings, whether it be a nearby national park, a forest, or any other wilderness area, research them beforehand. Find out which areas are most crowded and when. Avoid them when possible or at least avoid them during the busiest hours (usually it's the weekends). The most popular hiking trails don't always mean the best ones. Even if they do offer the most spectacular views, the diminished experience of admiring them with hundreds of people around you might not be worth it. A less frequented trail nearby can be a better alternative as long as it's accessible for your fitness level. If you can't find any viable options, consider a less popular natural area close to the one you wanted to visit. Some areas around the popular wilderness areas can be just as beautiful but don't come with crowds. For the purposes of enjoying the sense of open spaces, any quiet natural setting with expansive views will do.

You can also regain a sense of wide, open spaces by taking up hobbies that involve being in the water, particularly in the ocean. This includes surfing of all kinds, sailing, kayaking, scuba diving, and stand-up paddleboarding. For those who are allergic to plants, the ocean might be one of the only safe oases where they can connect with nature without suffering from uncomfortable symptoms.

If you don't live by a big body of water, depending on the area where you live, you can consider hobbies exposing you to wild open spaces that involve spending time:

- in the mountains (hiking, climbing, mountain biking, paragliding).
- in the desert (off-road expeditions, hiking, or horseback riding),
- in the forest or its waterways (bushcraft, rafting, birdwatching).

Here are the key actions you can take to avoid the negative effects of reduced access to wide, open spaces:

- Develop awareness of how often you spend time in crowded places and if it affects your mental health. If you feel uneasy when brushing shoulders with hundreds of people, avoid going to public venues when they're most crowded.

- Assess your commuting options. If possible, bike or walk to work instead of commuting in a crowded metro or a bus.

- Become your city's explorer. Seek quiet, safe places with few people around where you can enjoy some much-needed solitude outside of your home.

- Regularly look as far away as you can see, ideally in a natural setting. If you don't have access to any open spaces, take up skygazing instead.

- When exploring wild areas outside of your city—or even natural environments in an urban setting—seek least crowded trails and go during the least busy hours. You don't have to go to the most popular national park nearby. Sometimes lesser-known areas can be as beautiful.

- Take up outdoor hobbies exposing you to wide, open spaces. This includes water activities like surfing or sailing, mountain activities like climbing or mountain biking, desert activities like hiking or off-road driving, and forest activities such as bushcraft or birdwatching.

CHAPTER 14

How Fast Is Too Fast?

ৰ৲

For Anne, who lives in London, the day starts at 5 a.m. with a blaring alarm clock. If it weren't for the torturous device, she wouldn't be able to wake up, as each night she gets five hours of sleep. She can't afford to sleep in and can't afford to get enough sleep. There's too much to do.

But she doesn't have time in the morning to think about it. She gets up, rushes to the bathroom, where she takes a quick shower, puts on make-up, gets dressed while drinking coffee, and leaves. Breakfast? She'll grab a sandwich on the way to the Tube. Or maybe not. She can't afford to miss the train. Her day in the office goes by in a blur. It's already dark outside, and she still needs to go to the gym, go grocery shopping, and prepare a business report for tomorrow.

As she's falling asleep at midnight, she wonders why she's so exhausted all the time. She dreams of her upcoming one-week vacation, when she plans to finally rest a little. After she takes care of the backlog of household chores, of course.

This is a fictional story, but perhaps you can see yourself in this example or know someone who lives like that. In all busy, fast-paced cities around the world, there are millions of people living just like Anne. It's opposite to how our ancestors lived for hundreds of thousands of years.

Nature is slow and patient. Look at the timeline of our evolution. It's hard to grasp how much time has passed and how insignificant our lifespans are compared to the history of how our species came to be, let alone the entire world history.

The problem is we now live faster than ever before, and arguably faster than we were ever meant to. Urban settings are the opposite of nature, pace-wise: high-stimuli and fast-paced, in an endless frenzy. We want everything now. We scream, shout, and swear when we're stuck in traffic. We get annoyed when someone in front of us walks a little too slowly for our liking. We can't afford to stop and think. Every second counts in a bustling city. Nature lover or not, it's easy to fall victim to the allure of fast urban living. After all, the busier you appear, the more important you are (or so people like to think).

Is this just the biased observation of disgruntled city dwellers, or do we indeed live faster in urban areas?

Observation of 1,300 pedestrians at ten places in Australia and England suggest that pedestrians move more quickly in big cities than in small towns.[119] Walking speed isn't the perfect way to measure the pace of life, though. It's possible that larger cities have higher populations of younger people who walk faster and lower populations of the elderly who move more slowly.

Comparing how fast people walk today compared to the past could help us spot a potential trend, however. In 2006, psychologist Richard Wiseman and the British Council conducted an experiment measuring walking speed in cities around the world. It has shown that the pace of life back then was 10 percent faster than in the early 1990s when an identical experiment was conducted (though with only 70 pedestrians measured in each city, take these numbers with a grain of salt).[120] Because of the small sample, it's still not a perfect study. What if we measure the pace of life in a different way?

A study comparing the pace of life in 31 countries around the world focused not only on the average walking speed in downtown locations, but also the speed with which postal clerks completed a simple request and the accuracy of public clocks. They found out that the pace of life was significantly slower in undeveloped countries[121] with the fastest in highly urbanized Japan and Western Europe. As the saying goes, people in fast-paced countries have watches, while people in slow-paced ones have time.

It's difficult to measure the pace of life, given the many factors that influence it. Yet there's little doubt that life before the invention of the internet and smartphones was slower. We were less distracted without our favorite devices. Before these technological advancements, we could get bored. We could let our minds wander, sit still and do nothing. This is how we would recharge back then. Today, not so much. Plugged in all the time, everyone can reach us at every moment. If we have merely a spare second, we turn our faces and our thumbs toward the smartphone screen. Recharging is reserved for our devices, not for our minds that crave constant stimulation, not unlike an addict craving another dose of their poison of choice.

The frenetic, 24/7 pace of big cities can be exciting for some people. They thrive on all the stimulation, seemingly unbothered by a lack of proper rest. But the human body wasn't designed to operate at full efficiency all the time, day in, day out. Free time spent away from work, chores, education, and necessary activities such as eating and sleeping is crucial for us. Research shows that leisure is therapeutic. It affects physical, social, emotional, and cognitive health.[122] It impacts life satisfaction[123] and subjective well-being.[124]

We need unstructured time off to recharge. We had it for the majority of our human history. Today, the frantic atmosphere of a fast-paced city makes relaxation difficult. It's hard to slow down when everyone around you is in a rush. And the more you speed up your life in an effort to keep up, the more often you miss precious moments, and, in the end, the less joy you get. What's the point of living so fast that your days pass by like a blur?

Dr. Stephanie Brown, psychologist, addiction specialist, and the author of *Speed: Facing Our Addiction to Fast and Faster—and Overcoming Our Fear of Slowing Down*, points out that "Countless people want to slow down in every way, but they cannot, even when they vow they're going to change. They want to set limits on their technology use, they vow to 'cut back,' they promise to be more available and engaged with their families, but they do not change. This is addiction: you cannot go any faster, and you cannot slow down, even when you want to."[125] In an interview with the New York Times, Brown said: "It's like we're all in this addicted family where all this busyness seems normal when it's really harmful. There's this widespread belief that thinking and feeling will only slow you down and get in your way, but it's the opposite."[126]

To make matters worse, those addicted to the fast pace often carry the same attitude with them while they rest or go on vacation, supposedly to relax. There's an endless list of places to see and things to do. The goal isn't to slow down and recharge one's batteries. The mission is to squeeze as many activities in during the time off as possible. It's the antithesis of leisure.

This doesn't happen to busy CEOs alone, though. Even those otherwise enthusiastic about spending time in nature often spend more time taking pictures or posting them on social media than enjoying their time in the wilderness. If you don't believe me, find a nice comfortable spot in a place frequented by tourists. Observe how many of them stay there longer than the time needed to take a couple of pictures. The vast majority are gone in five minutes, with only a few taking in the place without any distractions.

The hard truth is that no matter how many natural attractions you see during your trip or how many pictures you post on social media, you won't be connecting with nature if you don't pause and contemplate it. Natural surroundings can change us through contemplating them. We don't let them impact us by crossing them off a list in the fastest time possible to squeeze in another sight on the same day. A busy travel agenda is another sign of our addiction to speed and yet another failure to enjoy the moment.

Is a rural life without crowds, traffic jams, advertisements vying for your attention at every corner, and other common, stimulating aspects of an urban environment the only answer to battle the speed epidemic? There's no denying that exposure to an environment where change happens slowly and where nature is patient can help. But speed addiction is contagious, no matter where you live. Urbanite or not, fast life is now so imbued in the modern society. Merely putting some physical distance between you and bustling cities might not be enough. The reason is in your pocket or maybe even your hand at this very moment. All it takes is to pull out your smartphone. What can we do to resist the distractions and breakneck pace of life and slow down a little? Let's explore some solutions.

CHAPTER 15

Solutions: Combatting the Crazy Pace of Living

ဆ

Slowing down starts in your mind. It's tempting to believe that the faster we move and the faster we act, the more we live. But do we live *better* if we rarely, if ever, take the time to pause and savor the present moment? Do our modern lives resemble the nature-infused lives of our ancestors in any way if even when we're out in the wilderness, we still think about our urban lives? Can we appreciate nature at all if we can't let go of our high-technology, high-pace lives for a moment and be still in the face of all the non-digital life around us?

To overcome this troubling tendency, practice mindfulness. Focus on whatever you're doing at the moment instead of planning your next move or multi-tasking. A good way to train this ability is to take a walk in natural surroundings and tune out all the distractions around you. Focus on the environment around you. Look at the features of the landscape and the small elements. Can you notice the complex texture of tree bark? Can you feel the rough surface of a rock? Can you spot the various shapes of the waves breaking on the beach? It sounds easy, but it's anything but for the average city dweller accustomed to distractions all around. And that's why it's such a valuable exercise to regain some control over your pace of life.

For me, one of the most powerful exercises to stay in the moment are sports with consequences. If you're surfing, you can't let your mind wander or you'll fall off your board or get hit by a wave you failed to see as you were thinking of something else. The high focus the sport requires is like training for the brain, and not just for the body.

Yoga and any other activity that employs balance and breathwork is yet another way to learn how to be still. The consequences of losing focus aren't as dramatic as when surfing, but the mechanism remains the same. You lose focus, you lose balance in a pose. You fail to breathe properly, you can feel your body getting tense (or failing to relax).

Strive to do less, but better, versus doing as much as you can without ever paying attention to what you're doing. Somewhat counterintuitively, a busy calendar makes us less productive. We spread ourselves too thin, and no task gets our full attention. Focus only on what's essential. If possible, delegate or disregard the rest so you have time for yourself. Say no more often so you can say yes to more valuable activities. Put space between tasks in your calendar so you don't spend the entire day running from one errand to another. A looser schedule will also let you be more spontaneous (how about a quick walk to a park or by the beach?).

When going on vacation or weekend trips, pay close attention to how you structure your days. If you're away from work, you're not supposed to create another job for yourself by creating a to-do list of things to see and activities to do. Allow at least some of the days to be spontaneous. Spend extended time at attractions you enjoy, but without wielding your phone. Be still and enjoy them as they are without worrying how they'll look on your timeline.

I used to travel with a detailed plan of where I wanted to go and what I wanted to see on each day. Thankfully, I've learned to travel less prepared and be more flexible. This way, I enjoy my trips more. I can connect with nature on a deeper level as I breathe in the views without checking the time or planning how to cross another attraction off my list. Some of my favorite travel memories now are of sitting still in beautiful natural surroundings. I wasn't doing anything special there. It was being out there without any particular plans in mind. Often, these places weren't mentioned in any guidebooks or top ten things to do.

Technology can be beneficial when we're out in nature, but it can ruin our already diminished attention. Develop a habit to silence at least some notifications on your phone when you're on a walk in a park or anywhere in nature. Few of us are ready to completely turn off our phones. So, how about silencing at least some of the notifications to reduce the distraction caused by never-ending beeps and dings?

My way of dealing with this is to disable Internet (both Wi-Fi and mobile data) on my phone. If I want to check something, I need to turn it on again. This way, I'm not constantly bothered by various notifications that make it difficult to be in the moment. At the same time, I'm still reachable if someone wants to call me or text me.

Lastly, a simple strategy to reduce your pace of life is to start your day slower. One of my favorite ways to reinforce a slower pace of life is to wake up early. No matter where in the world you are, even in a city that never sleeps, early mornings are the quietest period of the day with the fewest distractions. If you don't want to or can't wake up early, consider waking up at least 15 minutes earlier. This way, you'll start your day a little slower and set the right tone for the rest of the day.

Here are the key actions you can take to slow down:

- Slowing down starts with mindfulness. Tune out distractions and focus on the present moment.

- Keep your schedule a little looser to be able to spontaneously enjoy nature or enjoy a peaceful moment.

- Don't turn your vacations into yet another job. Be cautious not to plan every single day with a to-do list and an hourly schedule.

- When out in nature, silence at least some notifications on your phone so that your experience won't get interrupted every few minutes.

- Start your day slower by waking up a little earlier. Take the time to set the right, mindful tone for the rest of the day.

The best way to handle the problems associated with a fast pace of living and constant distractions everywhere we go is to find the balance between urban living and nature. Being constantly exposed to our bustling, urban environments where everything moves at breakneck speed, isn't good for our mental health. Meanwhile, even a simple act of sitting on a bench in a park and gazing at a tree can help us unwind. That brings us to the third part of the book. It's where we'll discuss how to achieve the proper balance: enjoying the benefits of modern living without giving up the blessings offered by nature.

PART 3

Finding the Balance Between Urban Living and Nature

Istanbul, Turkey is one of the most important cities in history. Founded under the name of Byzantion and later known as Constantinople, it served as a capital for some of the most powerful empires throughout history. These days, Istanbul enjoys the status of a global city and is one of the most popular tourist destinations in the world. But while the city can be proud of its human-centric accomplishments, its residents deal with a problem unknown for almost the entire length of our presence on Earth. They're hard-pressed to find any green spaces nearby, let alone anything resembling nature in its wild state.

Only 2.2 percent of Istanbul belongs to public green spaces.[127] One of the largest parks in the city, Emirgan Park, covers an area of 117 acres (470,000 square meters). It's seven times less than the area of Central Park. That's for a city which has almost double the population of New York. To further compare how inadequate green spaces are in Istanbul, New York's biggest park, Pelham Bay Park, is almost 24 times larger than Emirgan Park. There's just not enough nature in Istanbul to be available to everyone, and its residents have paid for it with blood.

In 2013, when the government announced plans to replace one of the last parks with a new urban development, peaceful environmentalists staged a sit-in protest. After a brutal police crackdown that included using tear gas, pepper spray, water cannons, and burning down the tents of the protesters, the protest turned nationwide. A woman wearing a red dress and standing her ground as she was being sprayed by a policeman became an iconic symbol of the protests. Millions of people across the country soon joined the demonstrations. Sadly, some died after being hit in the head with tear gas canisters and suffering other injuries. The situation got out of control. Protesters hijacked a bulldozer and chased police vehicles. The numbers of injured victims reached the thousands.

For the record, saying a lack of green spaces alone led to the protests would be a gross simplification. The construction plans and the government's reaction to the sit-in protest were the final straw in a country with a tense political situation. Environmental issues, including cutting down over 2.7 million trees for the construction of a new bridge and an airport, also played a role. Nonetheless, what initially sparked the pandemonium was a peaceful sit-in protest to protect one of the last green spaces in the city.

But let's not pick on one city. Cities around the world struggle with low access to green spaces. For example, only 3.4 percent of Taipei is reserved for public parkland. The futuristic city might have an impressive skyline, but its investment in nature leaves a lot to be desired. South American Bogotá dedicates 4.9 percent of its area to parks and gardens. You would think that in Colombia, a country known for its biodiversity, there would be more greenery in its capital. Unfortunately, that's not the case. The crowded megacity of Tokyo, one of the world's most important and powerful global cities, isn't generous to its residents either. It assigns just 7.5 percent of its area to public green spaces. But let's be honest: when you think of megalopolis of Tokyo, quiet green spaces are probably the last thing that come to mind.

So, let's move to Europe, home to the earliest urban parks in the world. It turns out that some of the most well-known cities in the old continent don't fare much better. The world's second most visited city, Paris, might offer iconic landmarks, but green spaces aren't as well-known. Just 9.5 percent of the city's area belongs to public parkland. Another popular European destination, Amsterdam, stands at 13 percent.

How about North American cities? In Austin, Texas, 11 percent of the city is allotted to public green spaces. In San Francisco, California, as well as in Toronto, in otherwise heavily forested Canada, it's 13 percent.

If we want a greener future, all these popular cities should be leading by example. Unfortunately, that's not the case. We could argue it's still a lot, given how expensive urban land is. But is it really that much considering how important nature is for our well-being?

Of course, there are also cities that have a respectable area dedicated to green spaces. Oslo dedicates a staggering 68 percent of its area for public green spaces. It's one of the reasons why it was named The European Green Capital of 2019. The city state of Singapore, despite limited space, doesn't make excuses as they pursue their goal of becoming a city in a garden. Currently, 47 percent of its area belongs to public green spaces. Other examples of green cities include Sydney with 46 percent of its area belonging to public parkland, Vienna with 45.5 percent, and Chengdu with 42.3 percent. Out of 37 cities studied by World Cities Culture Forum, the median percentage of public green space was 22 percent.[128]

It seems unavoidable for nature lovers to feel detached from nature in cities where almost 80 percent of the area is man-made. But let's not limit ourselves to defining nature by public green spaces alone. What about a general perception of greenery around us? Maybe a city doesn't have many parks, but it has so many tree-lined street trees that it gives an impression of living close to nature. There's a measure called Green View Index that calculates exactly that. Created by the MIT Senseable City Lab, the index analyzes the amount of green perceived while walking down the street, excluding public parks.[129]

Unfortunately, many of the world's leading cities still fare badly. Paris stands at a paltry 8.8 percent and scored the worst among 27 studied cities. London was calculated at 12.7 percent, New York City at 13.5 percent, Los Angeles at 15.2 percent, Toronto at 19.2 percent, and Amsterdam at 20.6 percent. The city with the highest Green View Index was Tampa, Florida, with 36.1 percent. But we don't all live in subtropical Tampa. The median score was 20 percent. This means that even using a measure taking into account street trees only, little nature surrounds most city dwellers.

Of course, not everyone is bothered. Some prefer concrete, metal, asphalt, glass, and plastic over trees, ocean waves, mountain peaks, wide open spaces, wetlands, and wildlife. There isn't anything wrong per se with those who enjoy urban environments and don't care much about spending time in natural surroundings. Not everyone has to be an outdoorsy person.

But those urbanites who do crave nature—people like you, for whom I wrote this book—are in a difficult spot. On one hand, cities provide convenience, opportunities, and a plethora of other benefits. On the other hand, as the numbers we discussed show, access to nature is limited in urban areas.

How can we find a compromise between living in a city and living close to nature? Can we even accomplish this lofty task? That's what we'll discuss in the third part of this book. But first, we need to answer one key question.

CHAPTER 16

What Does Connecting With Nature Mean in Today's Urbanized World?

ఎ.

To talk about a compromise between urban living and connecting with nature, we should define what connecting with nature means. That means we need to define "nature" first. It's not an easy task because nature is a word that has as many definitions as there are people to define it. If you read Wikipedia's article on nature, you'll see pictures of beautiful waterfalls, picturesque mountains, tropical coastlines, majestic old-growth forests, and oceans—but also outer space, lightning strikes, microscopic mites, and modern cities. Broadly speaking, nature is the entire universe. But this doesn't help us much if we want to define what "connecting with nature" means.

A more useful definition of nature would be describing it as the natural, wild environment. But as we've learned over the previous chapters, true wilderness, free of human interference or with very little human footprint, is rare in the modern world. The effects of our activity reach even the most-distant corners of the globe. Planes fly all over the planet, generating noise pollution even in the remotest areas. Trash reaches even the most far-flung desert islands. Were you to be stranded on one, you'd still be reminded civilization exists.

Also, we can't ignore the fact that today's wilderness areas haven't stayed unchanged for millennia. What is today a protected park visited for recreation, might have once accommodated seasonal shepherding that has shaped the landscape we see today. Or it might have been permanently inhabited by humans.

For example, consider the tragic example of Native Americans removed from their lands. Then there's also the impact of people and goods traveling across the world.

For example, Nā Pali Coast State Park on the island of Kauai in the Hawaii is a landscape that seems unchanged for centuries. However, it was in fact changed by humans through the introduction of invasive species, which has led to a struggle for local plants to survive. Non-native trees like eucalyptus release toxins into the soil. This discourages other plants from growing nearby. Without dense local vegetation, when it rains, water isn't absorbed and released into streams slowly. Instead, mud forms, leading to flash floods destroying endemic plants and posing damage to humans.[130] Eucalyptus might look like an innocent tree. To an untrained eye it looks like a member of native flora. Meanwhile, in fact, its introduction by humans dramatically changed the local landscape.

Joan Maloof, the director of forest conservation non-profit Old-Growth Forest Network, writes in her book *Nature's Temples: The Complex World of Old-Growth Forests* that "We don't even know what forests should look like anymore. Do we notice that the forest we are walking through has fewer herbaceous plants and fewer types of herbaceous plants than it had once upon a time? No, because we have likely never experienced a forest like that near our town. We don't even know what's possible."

Only the most remote destinations can be considered "true" wilderness areas that has remained largely free of human influence. They include the desolate Canadian Arctic Archipelago, the bear-friendly East Siberian taiga, the scorching hot Australian outback, the heart of the Amazon rainforest, or parts of the Sahara Desert.

But does connecting with nature need to be reserved for the affluent and adventurous only? Can we only experience the wonders of the natural world if it's untouched by humans? And is isolated, pristine wilderness the only land worthy of our protection and appreciation? What about our urban and suburban landscapes where we live and work? Don't they deserve that same care and attention?

As I went for a walk to an urban forest close to where I live, I saw a squirrel scurrying up a tree. It chirped to let me know it saw me as we gazed at each other. Then I saw a woodpecker drumming against the same tree higher in the canopy. It didn't like me being there and flew away.

Was my experience of connecting with nature inferior to that of watching the same wildlife in a national park? Isn't this pocket of urban nature worth respect and appreciation, too? True, I could also hear car traffic and see buildings. Nonetheless, I was *in* nature, even if it wasn't a pristine, quiet old-growth forest. Would I prefer to be able to wander through a primeval forest? Of course. Unfortunately, that's not possible where I live, so the next best thing is to enjoy what's available. Whenever I can, I travel to more remote natural areas. In my everyday life, I take what I can. A city-dwelling nature lover needs to find a compromise. Daily natural exposure in small doses is preferable to taking the view that only being out in the wilderness can constitute a true experience of connecting with other life forms.

For context, in Poland, where I live, until 2019 it wasn't even legal to spend a single night in any of the state forests. It was only legal to do so in a designated place, usually by a road or a dirt parking lot—not in nature. And these forests aren't even pristine old-growth forests. I would define them more as managed plantations due to a pine-dominated landscape, crisscrossed with wide access roads.

But even now that bivouacking in certain forests is possible as long as visitors respect certain rules, the forests in my region—or anywhere in the country for that matter—don't offer many opportunities to get away from civilization. For example, I used Google satellite view to find how far away I could get from the nearest settlements and paved roads in the largest forest in the country that allows wild camping. The "wildest" place I could find was about six kilometers (four miles) away from the closest road. In flat terrain, that's an hour-long casual walk. And we're not talking about a dense, old-growth forest full of life where you can get lost. It's a young, managed forest planted in rows, often with grassy access roads between them.

Wilder areas do exist in Poland—primarily in the mountains—but even there, you won't get away from other people. Wild camping is prohibited and most camping grounds are crowded in the season. Moreover, these less populated areas are still by no means remote like the largest wilderness areas in the U.S. or even some parks in Europe. If you're looking for wild nature a considerable distance away from civilization, you won't find it in Poland.

And yet, here I am, a nature lover in a country with virtually non-existent access to wild areas who somehow manages to stay sane (it's not always easy, mind you). That's why I understand the struggles of fellow city-dwelling nature lovers. And that's why I decided to title this book *Connecting with Life*. I propose to define nature as every landscape that hosts life—whether it's an undeveloped coastline, or a copse of trees, or a stretch of rolling prairies, or a public green space. Even a potted plant can provide us with the enjoyment of connecting with another form of life.

If we limit the definition of connecting with nature to extraordinary experiences, we'll turn it into a privilege limited to few people. This is the total opposite of what nature should be. The poor and the rich, the fit and the less fit, the adventurers and the homebodies—nature can and should be accessible to and enjoyed by all. One nature lover might get, if you will, a stronger kick from a weeklong expedition to the Siberian taiga but it doesn't mean that a simple walk down an urban park of another nature lover is something to be scoffed at. Connecting with nature shouldn't be degraded to yet another pointless exercise in one-upping people. We want as many people as possible experiencing the natural environment in whatever form it is accessible to them so that we all care for the planet.

When we think of nature as something untamed, pristine, and untouched, we set such high expectations that we fail to see the beauty in the prosaic, daily encounters in the small pockets of our cities or our backyards. Each time a bird lands on the balcony of my apartment—whether it's the Eurasian jay, the great tit, the black and white Eurasian magpie, or even the common wood pigeon—I feel awe (particularly when the bird stares back at me). I'm aware it might sound bizarre, if not outright absurd, to some readers. However, if we discount such experiences, we detach ourselves from nature through our own fault, not because we live in an urbanized world. Seeing the wonder in simple, fleeting moments is our own choice. Why not appreciate what's at our fingertips?

Environmental historian William Cronon argues in his article "The Trouble with Wilderness: Or, Getting Back to the Wrong Nature" that we need to "embrace the full continuum of a natural landscape that is also cultural, in which the city, the suburb, the pastoral, and the wild each has its proper place, which we permit ourselves to celebrate without needlessly denigrating others."[131]

This is the theme that we'll explore in more detail in the next few chapters as we go through the various strategies to connect with nature daily. The second part of the book is heavy on scientific research, statistics, and other facts. Here, we'll get a bit more philosophical (don't worry, we'll still discuss practical suggestions).

As Marcus Aurelius wrote in his *Meditations*, "Life itself is but what you deem it." So is bonding with nature and life in itself: it starts in our minds and how we perceive the world around us. Whether we live in the city or in the countryside, we first need to adopt a philosophy that will help us see and appreciate what's around us. This is both about tiny doses of nature as well as its most majestic manifestations.

That's not to say that we should stop caring about the wild areas and conform with their disappearance because hey, these urban birds can be cool, too. Making a choice to see nature even in the urban settings will help us stay connected to it. This will then encourage us to conserve, protect, and grow it. Ultimately, we'll learn to appreciate the miracle of life whatever form it takes. This will make us even more appreciative of our national parks and reserves, state forests, and other natural environments.

To see some examples of nature in cities, visit my website at *www.MartinSummerAuthor.com* and access bonus book resources. The password is "connecting."

CHAPTER 17

Getting Mindful:
Learning to Pay Attention

2&

As I think of city-dwelling nature lovers, I imagine someone like me who doesn't need encouragement to spend time in natural environments whenever possible. But "whenever possible" is the key word here. Our modern, urbanized world has gifted us many conveniences but also many new responsibilities. Living and working in the city can make it difficult to engage in frequent, meaningful exposure to nature. It's hard to get out into nature for several hours, let alone several days. But as we've explored in the previous chapters, that doesn't mean we're destined to live a life of deprivation. We don't have to be detached from nature because we want to enjoy the conveniences of city living.

Let's explore various ways to interact with nature daily and/or make each interaction deeper. None of the following ideas require a lot of time, money, long-term commitments (that's why as incredible as having a pet can be, this way of bonding with nature isn't included in this chapter), or any other resources. The goal is to combat and avoid feeling detached from nature by learning how to inject it into your everyday urban life. When you pair these daily strategies with day trips, weekend trips, or longer vacations in natural environments, you'll start feeling closer and more connected to nature.

First, let's focus on step one: paying attention.

The other day I sat with my girlfriend at the edge of a small forest 20 minutes away from where we live. As we enjoyed the blue skies and the feeble warmth of the February sun, a woodpecker landed on a thick branch no more than 20 feet away (six meters). It started drumming the tree in search of its next meal. Perhaps we were quiet enough for its liking, or perhaps it didn't care about our presence. Either way, we had front row seats to watch its methodical, skilled work. And we did for the next 20 minutes as it stripped the bark, making high-pitched noises, hammering countless holes in the branch. It was an unexpected spectacle on an otherwise normal day. We participated in it only because we paid attention. We enjoyed it only because we learned to appreciate the little things.

I haven't always been so attentive and aware of nature. I used to discount its value because it wasn't anything exotic or truly "wild" (whatever the term means). But if we can't appreciate nearby nature even when surrounded by concrete and asphalt, can we appreciate nature in general? Do we need a checklist to identify which experiences of connecting with life are "valid" and which ones don't count because there was, say, a man-made structure in sight? I'd argue that any encounter, as long as it's meaningful to you (and only you can choose whether it is or isn't), is valuable.

Then there's the elephant in the room: our tendency to keep ourselves distracted all the time, struggling to focus on a single thing even for a few minutes. How are we supposed to notice tiny birds hiding in the trees or more elusive forms of life if most of the time we're checking our phones, planning the day ahead, reflecting on the past, or doing any other tasks than actually focusing on the present moment? Dr. Stephanie Brown, the author of *Speed* (who we've already met when we discussed fast urban living), emphasizes on her blog that one of the key mantras she restates throughout her book is: "Pause, ask yourself 'what am I doing?' Take a breath. Reflect. Without a working capacity for, and value of, self-reflection, we truly abdicate self-responsibility."[132]

This simple exercise, repeated daily at least a few times, is like mental training that will bring your wandering mind back to the present moment. Make it a habit to regularly ask yourself what you're doing. Do so particularly when you're exposed to nature, even if it's a small urban park or when you're walking by a body of water. Place your feet firmly into this moment: not what you're going to do today or tomorrow or what you did yesterday or what this or that person said about you. Leave it for now and participate in life as it unfolds at this very moment.

The river that runs through my city isn't of particular beauty, but if you pause and look for a second, you can see fascinating patterns caused by wind. You can see the currents and how fast the objects disappear when caught in them. You can even see some wildlife like ducks or seagulls. It's mind-blowing how in recent years so many of the latter have adapted to the urbanizing world by moving to inland cities. Experts say that rural gulls are in massive decline while the number of urban gulls is rapidly increasing and expected to continue going up.[133]

On my various trips, I also strive to focus on what's around me, regardless if it's a built-up, semi-natural, or wild area. I appreciated local birds in a small park in Phoenix, Arizona. On hikes throughout the Spanish and Greek countryside, I enjoyed passing local goats and sheep. I was happy to spot otters crossing a park in Singapore with dozens of people around. A seal checked me out with curiosity as I surfed in the frigid Baltic Sea in winter on a less developed part of the coastline—and I loved every moment of it. In the same way, though in warm turquoise waters of urbanized Freights Bay in Barbados, I loved surfing among turtles. An encounter with green monkeys running across the road in the less developed part of the island—something which, objectively speaking, doesn't sound like a big deal considering how many of them populate the island and how often you see them—was also a memorable experience.

And so was seeing another animal regularly crossing the island's roads: a mongoose. There's an interesting story behind their presence on the island. They were introduced to eradicate rats that ravaged sugar cane plantations. The plan failed because the mongoose hunted snakes during the day while the rats feasted in the sugar cane fields at night. Very few snakes can now be found on the island. Exploring the stories behind animals you encounter daily can be an excellent way to develop a deeper understanding and connection with nature.

These are all just a few examples of simple, but powerful encounters with life in both urban and less-developed areas. They all provided a feeling of connection and happiness because I chose to let them make me feel those emotions.

If we only allow ourselves to feel joy during the rare moments of exhilaration, say, when getting married or during childbirth, we lose the everyday beauty.

Interacting with nature works in the same way. It starts with our presence and our choice, not our environment. The ability to contemplate what's happening around us at the present moment—not pondering the past or planning the future—is closely associated with how much we can—or cannot—enjoy the natural surroundings. After all, even the most glorious wild areas won't provide any real, lasting feeling of connection to people busy snapping pictures and posting them on social media.

Whether we pay attention or not is within our responsibility. The cities where we live might not offer world-class natural wild environments. But a keen mind will find beauty and connection with nature when another will fail to see anything except for the screen of their smartphone. Urban life does exist if you only let yourself see it. Spotting it might not be as easy as in a pristine biodiverse Costa Rican rainforest. It doesn't mean that living in a city or a highly-urbanized country precludes you from connecting with animals and other life forms, though.

We miss a lot when we don't pay attention to what's around us. But even when we're attentive, we can still miss things—out of ignorance or a lack of awareness. This lack of knowledge also detaches us from the natural world and its wonders that are often hiding in plain sight. As I've explained it in the previous chapter, Poland can't boast about its wild areas. For a long time, I also assumed that it's devoid of much wildlife. Much of the non-urban areas of the country is farmland where little life can find refuge. Meanwhile, many forests are monocultural, failing to provide for a wide variety of species. Of course, compared to the most biodiverse countries in the world, it's indeed a poor place to see animals in the wild. But they're still there. You just have to educate yourself on their behavior and look a little closer to find the signs of their activity. You can apply the same approach wherever you live.

For example, I sometimes go on a walk by ponds that used to be filled with peat. In the last century, local inhabitants excavated them to collect peat as a fuel source. Today, they're used for retention and fire protection. It all sounds terribly boring and devoid of wildlife, yet if you look closely, you can notice countless signs of beaver activity. Learning more about those elusive animals, even if I've yet to see them out in the wild, provides a feeling of connection with nature through understanding how the species live. Then there are various frogs, birds, and wetland flora. The ponds are a mere few minutes away from a busy road. Yet, if you make an effort to educate yourself about them, you can experience a deep connection with nature. That's despite the area not being, objectively speaking, anything special, if not outright ugly and untidy to some.

Take a closer look at similar areas in or near your city and educate yourself about their history and the fauna and flora you can find there. Maybe you won't be able to spot all the inhabitants or you'll fail to see anything. Yet connecting with other forms of life by seeking the signs of their activity can be still a rewarding experience. It doesn't require any resources on your part other than the willingness to learn.

Learn how to identify the tracks of various animals. Listen to recorded bird calls. Memorize the ones you hear most often. Then try to differentiate between them as you're out in nature. Learn about different types of rock, bark, and soil. Touch them as you're out in nature to feel their unique texture. Discover the reason behind common natural smells and seek them out. For example, pine trees smell good because they release pinene and limonene into the air when they're damaged. Learn about edible foods available in your local area and, if possible, taste them out in the wild.

The Japanese practice of *shinrin-yoku*, or forest bathing, originated in the country in the 1980s. It's now regarded as one of the most well-researched forms of nature therapy. As the name implies, it's about bathing in the forest atmosphere through using all your senses. By being in nature and opening your senses to it—without participating in any other activities like hiking or jogging—you let the forest into your mind where it works its restorative magic.

When seeking encounters with nature, strive to make the experience more immersive by using as many senses as possible. How do you do that? Let's discuss it over the next chapters!

CHAPTER 18

The Art of Using Our Senses: How to See

ࢠ

The more senses we use to interact with nature, the richer the experience is. This doesn't change whether you're in an urban park, on a beach, in a national park, sitting under a tree, or in an armchair in your backyard watching the sunset. This also doesn't change for those who can't use all their senses because of hearing or vision loss, or other impairments. Nature can and should be enjoyed equally by everyone through a variety of senses. Using as many senses as you can will boost your enjoyment of nature and make each experience more memorable and, by extension, more beneficial, too. Over the next five chapters we'll discuss how to boost your enjoyment of nature through employing your senses more deeply.

Let's discuss sight first. We've already discussed how important it is to pay attention when we're in natural surroundings. If we're distracted, we might look, but we won't *see* what's around us. Sometimes when I'm on a forest walk with a friend and we have a deep conversation, an hour later I find myself realizing that I might have been to a forest, but I haven't seen it. It was a blurry background for our chat. This doesn't have to be bad—after all, I met with a friend to talk with him and pay attention to what he's saying, not the trees around. But this example shows how easy it is to be *physically* in a natural environment but *mentally* somewhere else. In the same way, even on a simple walk in the city, if we don't pay attention, we won't notice all the little manifestations of nature around. We won't notice street trees, urban wildlife, clouds with interesting shape, sunsets, etc.

Experiencing the natural surroundings by yourself can make it easier to see, but a willing nature-loving partner (a friend, a significant other, a relative) can point out things we would otherwise miss. The key word is, yet again, *attention*. One helpful technique, described in Tom Brown Jr.'s memoir *The Tracker*, is known as "splatter vision." It's about letting your vision spread out, not focusing on anything in particular, to become more sensitive to movement. When you notice movement, you focus on the object. According to *Princeton University Outdoor Action Guide to Nature Observation & Stalking* by Rick Curtis, "Focused vision doesn't pick up movement whereas wide-angle vision makes the eye reactive to movement."[134]

When I'm in a forest and hear a woodpecker drumming on a tree, I often pause and try to pinpoint its location. Tree by tree, canopy by canopy, branch by branch, I glance in many directions until I eventually notice a tiny movement. It's difficult, if not outright impossible, to locate the bird without my eyes sweeping around. Come to think of it, I usually spot a woodpecker out of the corner of my eye, masked so well that if it wasn't moving, there would be no way to notice it.

In the city there might also be wildlife we don't see because we're focused on a specific object versus letting our vision spread out. Wherever in the world you are, animals are often hiding in plain sight. My girlfriend and I spotted a koala in Noosa National Park in Australia while dozens of people missed it because they didn't know where to look. And it was right above them!

When we lived in Barbados, we spotted green monkeys in rural areas. They were brought in the late 17th century on slave ships from West Africa. The rural monkeys prefer to watch you hidden from a long distance. It's a fun game to spot them. Curiously, the ones living in more urban settings don't mind being seen or outright challenging humans (including stealing from them).

Seeing all this wildlife is only possible when you choose to focus on this task, not on merely looking around while you think about something else. As a side note, visit my website at *www.MartinSummerAuthor.com* to see pictures of some of the locations mentioned throughout this book. The password is "connecting."

In addition to looking *at* things, it's important to look *through* things, too. For example, that tree right in front of you might partly block your view, but you can still see through the branches and through its leaves. That's where an animal might be hiding. In the city, this might mean looking through the canopy of a street tree that might host some wildlife like a bird's nest or a squirrel.

During your outing, pick one thing to focus on. For example, if you're heading for a quick walk in an urban park, you can decide to watch the behavior of one species of local birds alone, e.g. ducks. How do they move? How do they communicate with each other? How do they differ in appearance? It's like having your private *Planet Earth* moment—as long as you give yourself at least a few minutes to sit still and observe. In the same way, you can focus on spotting a specific local flower or plant or on learning how to identify different species by leaves or bark. We've discussed how educating yourself can help you enjoy nature more. Use your sight to become a local nature expert.

When we speak of sight, we should also re-emphasize the importance of looking at all the distances if possible. This isn't always easy in an urban setting, but usually you can look out at the horizon from a bridge or a public waterfront space. Tall structures will also do, particularly if at least a portion of the view is over a natural landscape, like the coast or an urban park.

Look at what's right below you or near you, too. For example, be conscious of where you step, particularly on a dirt path. When hiking, I sometimes like to tune out everything around me except for the trail under my feet and the next step I'm going to take. It feels like meditation that, in a way, connects me with the ground. I don't see what's around me and above me, but I do see some new things on the ground that I would have otherwise missed.

Look at the small details of various natural objects, too. Have you ever picked up a leaf to see its texture from up close? Can you tell the difference between two species of trees? When I was planting a small forest in my parents' backyard, some saplings weren't labeled. They looked so similar to each other that it seemed impossible to identify them. After consulting Google, I learned that the leaves of one tree species had tiny hairs while the other didn't. Leaf by leaf, each inches from my face, I managed to spot the difference. A difficult challenge turned into a rewarding and educational experience.

Have you ever observed an insect walking on your arm? Have you ever noticed how sharp and eroded wind-exposed cliffs are? This type of mindfulness might sound woo-woo, but there doesn't have to be anything spiritual about it. It's a reminder to become more aware of all the little ways in which nature is interwoven in our daily lives. That's even if it's just a leaf falling from a tree that you then rake to keep your backyard neat and tidy (and, with hope, use the leaves for compost).

Lastly, change your perspective by lying down on the grass, sand, a rock, or even an uneven forest floor. Use it as an opportunity to admire the sky above you (something you might have not done since childhood). Or observe the micro-life of insects, an ignored-by-many aspect of the natural world. Do you know that beetles account for 25 percent of all 1.5 million described species?[135]

Speaking of perspectives, have you ever noticed that an out-and-back trail looks different on a return trip? The trail hasn't changed, but your perspective has. A local urban park will also look different if you go in a different direction than usual (for example, clockwise instead of counterclockwise). A natural setting will also look different depending on the time of the day. Early mornings have a different vibe than afternoons or evenings. The time of the year (seasons) makes a difference, too, as well as weather (rainy, sunny, humid, dry). Mix up your outings to see the world—yes, including your local urban park—in a variety of ways. One beautiful example of this variety is the ocean. It can be tranquil and flat one day, choppy and angry the next, and then glassy, with perfect sets of waves coming in regular intervals (a surfer's dream). Then there are also tides, type and quality of waves, direction and strength of wind, and so many other things that make observing the ocean (ideally on a surfboard or while swimming) one of my favorite pastimes.

CHAPTER 19

The Art of Using Our Senses: Seek the Sounds

୬

Hearing is the next sense we use when exposed to nature. The world would be a sad place without birds singing, bees buzzing as they collect nectar, squirrels scuttling up a tree, crickets chirping on a hot summer evening, frogs croaking in a pond, or owls hooting at night. And what about waves crashing onto the beach, wind howling in a rugged mountainous terrain, or a stream burbling in the distance? Sadly, we often miss many of those sounds as we go about our business. Then we complain there's no nature around us.

Stop, pause, and seek the natural sounds around you as if you were hunting for them. Even in a city, there are many more sounds than just the artificial ones (although the man-made sounds do sometimes drown out the natural ones). For more focused hearing, cup your hands around your ears. This technique amplifies sounds and lets you hear a little better. Pushing your ears out is another strategy to better capture sound waves. It's like transforming your average-hearing human ears into vigilant deer ears (if you're afraid of judgment, try these techniques in a more secluded place).

One fun exercise I like to do to pay more attention to the sounds around me is to try to walk as silently as possible in any quiet, natural environment. As you avoid making noise, you become hyper-vigilant to any sources of noise around you. This makes it a great exercise in becoming more aware of your surroundings. Another option is to stop moving at all. When walking, all the shuffling or leaves crunching under your feet might mask what's going on around you. Stop, close your eyes if you feel comfortable, and become still for a few minutes. There's often a richness of sounds in the background we don't pick up on because we're too distracted or because the wildlife falls silent in response to the noise we're creating.

When we're out in nature, we often default to being active. We're walking, running, riding a bike, climbing, etc. As enjoyable as these activities can be, they make it difficult, if not outright impossible, to hear the wildlife around us. Startled by our noisy entrance into their world, the animals stay quiet until the danger passes. If we remain still for a few minutes, the sounds of nature might return—sounds we would otherwise never hear as we clang, crunch, and clomp. If you can't hear anything in particular, that's okay, too. Silence is a part of nature, as well. The last time I went to a forest for a listening session, I could hear birds only for the first few minutes when the sun was out. As it disappeared behind the clouds, the forest fell quiet, with the subtle sound of wind and creaking trees providing the only soundtrack.

As you head to a natural environment to listen to its sounds, don't make your first session too long. Sitting still and listening seems like an easy task, but in reality it's exhausting. It might even get frustrating as you find yourself getting distracted every few minutes. Our modern, stimulating world has made it difficult to engage in such meditative practices. Start small with a five- or ten-minute session. Make each one longer only when you feel comfortable.

Weather has a great impact on the sounds you can hear in nature. For example, I like listening to the creaking trees. There's even a word used to describe the melody of the wind in the trees: psithurism. A friend who rarely goes to forests was terrified by the sound as we went for a walk during a windy day. I find it soothing as I realize how many years of adverse conditions the trees have survived, and how they are still standing and still growing. Depending on its strength, wind can make a variety of noises in nature, from quiet rustling to loud blowing. Exploring nature during a hurricane might not be the safest way to enjoy natural sounds, though, so consider limiting oneself to manageable conditions.

Seasons can make a dramatic difference to the sounds you can hear in nature, too. In Poland in the summer forests are full of life. I get giddy just thinking about it. In the winter, everything goes silent and carries a depressive note (no, I'm not a fan of winters). The only exception is if there's snow, which adds a distinctive, muffled quality.

Regardless of the season, mornings sound different than afternoons. Afternoons sound different than nights. As a side note, if you want to listen to the night sounds, make sure to find a place where it's safe to do so first. Unfortunately urban parks are often not a good place to hang around when it's dark. In the tropics, sunset and sunrise sounds are particularly distinctive with all the animals announcing the beginning or the end of the day loud and clear.

Listening to the sounds of nature when you're in a public green space can be more difficult due to the surrounding man-made sounds. Is there any way we can handle this challenge? The first solution is to visit it during a quieter time of the day or week if you can—in the morning, early evening, or on the weekends, where there's less road traffic. To find your own secluded spot, seek quiet corners, perhaps less obvious or less attractive places. For example, seek areas without a flat patch of nice grass or places that can only be accessed via a muddy trail.

If you can't find a place free of constant man-made noises, try to tune out those sounds as you focus on what's around you. I like to think of it like two lovers in a crowd. There might be hundreds of strangers around them, but to them, none of those people exist. They're laser-focused on each other. We might not be able to completely tune out the unwanted sounds, but we can choose to focus on the nearby desirable sounds instead of obsessing over unwanted sounds we can't eliminate. Seeking natural white noise—such as that made by waves crashing on a beach, a fountain, or strong wind—is a neat trick to find some peace even in a busy city as it will help mask the man-made sounds.

If you find it hard to find tranquil natural areas in your city, you can turn your home into a little oasis by playing natural sounds on your speakers. You can't always go to the beach to listen to the waves or head to a forest to listen to the birds. But thanks to modern technology, you can still listen to them 24/7 if you want. Of course, it's not the real thing, but I still find it pleasant and relaxing to put some natural sounds in my earbuds and tune out the sounds of the city as I work.

Lastly, you don't always have to seek out sounds. The endless clamor that defines so many cities around the world isn't natural to humans. It's wise to seek some silence, too. For that, you don't even have to leave your house. Close all the windows, put your phone on silent, and perhaps use noise-blocking headphones or earplugs to give yourself a few minutes of peace. Even if all that surrounds you is concrete and asphalt, a few quiet minutes will help you reconnect with your decidedly much quieter roots.

CHAPTER 20

The Art of Using Our Senses: Smell the Roses (and Much More)

ða

Let's move on to the next sense: smell. Compared to seeing and hearing, it seems that we can't experience nature as deeply using our noses. After all, compared to most animals, we don't have a particularly strong sense of smell. But the reality is slightly different. Research conducted by John McGann, a neuroscientist at Rutgers University in New Jersey, shows that we have a similar number of olfactory bulb neurons to that of other mammals—including rodents and dogs.[136]

This doesn't mean that we have the same smelling ability, but it does suggest that with practice and attention, we can get much better than we think. Professional perfumer Sarah McCartney has spent 20 years learning to recognize different aromas. In her article for the Guardian, she says: "If you do want to improve your sense of smell, just practice. Pay more attention; smell the roses, the coffee, everything you eat and drink. If you smell something nice, stop and identify the source. You're probably already better at it than you imagine—and perhaps at least as good as your four-legged friends."[137]

This is the starting point to use our sense of smell more often in nature— through developing more awareness of the aromas around the house and in the cities where we live. With consistent daily practice, we'll start noticing more smells and get better at discerning them. The next time we're out in nature, we'll have a richer experience, too, as we start noticing things we haven't perceived before. Yes, there's a common theme here. By training our senses through becoming more mindful of what surrounds us, we build up our ability to more fully enjoy nature.

The type and strength of smells you can experience in nature often depends on weather: hot or cold, humid or dry, windy or calm. For example, one of the natural smells I enjoy the most is petrichor, the earthy scent produced when rain falls on soil after a long, warm, dry period. Curiously, the scent is stronger after light rain than after a heavy downpour. An organic compound responsible for this smell is geosmin, an earthy flavor and aroma produced by certain bacteria. Geosmin is also responsible for the earthy taste of beetroots. Some scientists believe that we are so sensitive to this smell because our ancestors relied on rainy weather for their survival.[138] It's yet another part of our inner wiring that hasn't gone away despite modern abundance. The next time there's rain after a dry spell, head outside to a public green space and enjoy this aroma.

Another distinct natural smell is the smell of ozone produced during a thunderstorm. When there's a storm coming, head outside before it starts to rain, and try to smell it. Wind from an approaching storm carries the ozone down from the clouds. An attentive observer will perceive the distinct smell in their nostrils.

Those blessed to live by the ocean or sea have daily access to one of the most characteristic natural smells: that of saltwater. Or, more precisely, something less romantic. It's a combination of dimethyl sulphide, produced by bacteria as they digest dead phytoplankton; dictyopterenes, sex pheromones produced by seaweed eggs to attract the sperm; and bromophenols produced by marine worms and algae.[139] The sources might not be as glamorous as we'd like. Yet, the unmistakable smell is still one we're drawn to and one that relaxes us. For many addicted to water sports, it's one that makes us jittery with excitement.

Seasons affect our ability to smell to a large extent. Winter is the poorest in scents because odor molecules move much more slowly as the air temperature drops. Moreover, according to Pamela Dalton, an olfactory scientist at the Monell Chemical Senses Center in Philadelphia, our noses don't work quite as well when the ambient air is cold because the olfactory receptors "bury themselves a little more deeply in the nose in winter" (possibly to protect against cold, dry air).[140] To cope with the deprivation of smells in winter, you can use an essential oil diffuser to fill your home with your favorite natural scent. You can also burn scented candles. To avoid indoor pollution caused by burning paraffin, use only natural candles such as those made of beeswax or soy wax. Make sure that wicks are made of cotton and that no synthetic oils, dyes, or scents are used in the candle. All the materials that make a candle are released into the air you breathe, so go natural.

On the other side of the spectrum, high temperatures and humidity on summer days affect bacteria growth. This makes smells stronger and more prevalent. Residents of big cities like New York or San Francisco can attest that their cities smell different (unfortunately, often worse) during the summer. Urban planner Victoria Henshaw said in her interview for NBC News that "the combination of heat and humidity allows bacteria to grow faster and smells to travel farther. The air becomes a smelly soup that we all breathe in."[141]

While intense city scents in the summer might not be exactly pleasant, warm weather also intensifies natural smells. This makes it the best period to hang out in a public green space or any natural area in search of new and old favorite scents: blossoming flowers, damp earth, freshly-mown grass, or woody forest aromas.

Whenever you're outdoors enjoying natural surroundings, do stop and smell the roses (or whatever other fragrance is available). Rub small bits of nature in your hand, like a pinch of soil, a dry leaf, or a flake of bark that fell off a tree. If it's been a long time since you last smelled any of those natural scents up close, you might find they bring back the added bonus of beautiful childhood memories. I don't know about you, but as a kid I sure loved getting all dirty and smelly because of all the mud, soil, grass, and no one knows what else I was covered in. To this day, I love the smell of earth.

CHAPTER 21

The Art of Using Our Senses: Can You Taste Nature?

ஆ

If you didn't consider smell as useful for natural exposure purposes as other senses we discussed, then taste is completely useless for getting a deeper connection with the natural world. After all, we don't go around the forest licking tree bark. We don't taste the flavor of sand on different beaches. And we most certainly don't try to drink unfiltered water from an unknown body of water in an effort to feel close to nature. But this doesn't mean that we can't use the sense of taste when we're in a natural environment. It might not be as easy as looking or hearing. However, with some effort or creativity we can taste nature—or use the sense of taste to make our natural outings more enjoyable.

The most obvious and perhaps most banal way to boost our enjoyment of being outside through using the sense of taste is to have a drink or eat in a natural setting. Before you say "duh," consider this—many activities that we do indoors are, at least for us nature lovers, more enjoyable outdoors. It's one thing to run on a treadmill and completely another to jog in a local park or down the beach. It's the same activity, but it feels different. In the same way, when you're on a hike in nature on a cold day, a hot beverage tastes like heaven. It's the same drink as the one you drink at home, but you enjoy it more—and along with the drink, you enjoy time spent outside more, too.

Whether it comes from the environment around you (pine-needle tea, anyone?) or not doesn't matter. The act of tasting *something* while exposed to nature will make the experience more vivid. Likewise, a picnic on the grass adds a new quality to what would otherwise be another walk in a park. Of course, this isn't often related to nature in itself. Water tastes better when we're on a strenuous hike, and fruits are fresher when we're having a day off, relaxing with our loved ones. But still—the more immersive your experience in nature is, regardless of the reason, the more enjoyable and memorable the activity is.

If you don't like my line of thinking, let's focus on tasting what comes directly from the natural surroundings around you. I'm always thrilled when I can eat some wild berries, while my parents are ecstatic to forage for wild mushrooms. Unfortunately, public green spaces rarely offer the opportunity to find edible food. This pastime is limited to those who have access to more expansive urban forests or other wilderness areas close or within the city limits.

Then there's also the issue of safety when wild foraging. When in doubt, always choose *not* to taste a berry, mushroom, or anything else you're unsure is edible. Hiring a local survival guide or joining a wilderness course to help you identify edible plants is one way of safely interacting with nature through taste. Reading a book on edible plants in the region could be a more affordable alternative as long as you're confident in your abilities to differentiate between various plants (again, when in doubt, don't eat). Don't forget that the foods you forage in the wild are eaten by the wildlife, too. Animals need it more than we do, which is why it's best to think of foraging as sampling nature rather than stuffing yourself.

Another way to use taste during our interactions with nature is to head to what I like to call "semi-natural" environments. They include: farms, orchards, vineyards, and gardens (all four ideally organic). Yes, you're in a man-made area. It's one rich in nature, though, even if it's managed, with crops and trees growing in neat rows. There's a whole lot you can taste depending on where and when you go: local wine, cheese, bread, fruits, vegetables, honey, etc. And often you don't have to head far away. A day trip may suffice to enjoy some tasty bits of nature.

Some farmers also let visitors pick fruit. To some, it might be a ludicrous pastime of city dwellers detached from nature. If you approach the farmers with respect for their hard work, though, you'll enjoy eating fresh produce picked by yourself and interact with people making a living off their relationship with nature. Agrotourism is an excellent way of understanding the joys and the struggles of going back to the land and working with one's hands. Scott Cohen, a professor of tourism management at the University of Surrey, in England, says in an interview for the Atlantic that: "Along with desk jobs can come a sense of disconnection from nature, and I think this is playing in. It allows for a tactile connection with nature. The 'work' is multi-sensual—one doesn't just see, but can smell, feel and taste the apples."[142] See? It's all about using multiple senses.

If there are no such opportunities near where you live, look into urban farming communities in your city. For example, on the edge of Oslo's city center (a city with a population of more than 650,000 people) you can find Losæter. It's an experimental urban farm, attracting students, herbalists, bakers, beekeepers, farmers, and volunteers of all kinds. Sitting between a highway and a trendy waterfront district, this thriving farm features row crops belonging more to the countryside than the capital city. There's also a serenity garden where residents of Oslo can find some peace. The farm even has a facility for baking with local grains. Everyone is welcome to help grow food—and enjoy a communal dinner afterward.[143] I can hardly think of a better way to have a good meal and interact with nature and the local community at the same time.

In the United States, there's a growing number of community gardens. Some provide affordable or free access to those who can't have a garden. These gardens are usually located on vacant land, school grounds, churches, and in senior centers, in cities both small and big. For gardens that require a paid membership, there's often a waitlist for plots. In some cases, while you wait, it's possible to contribute by helping with common projects or helping others with their plots.

In the United Kingdom, community gardens are often run by non-profits. For example, Fifth Quarter, a Norwich-based community group, describe themselves on their website in the following way: "Membership is open to anyone interested. Our oldest member is 84 and the youngest, 4. We provide everything needed—gardens, tools, seeds, a laugh—you provide time and interest... seems a fair deal. The gardens are run by volunteers and all produce is free to those who want it."[144] London also has community gardens. One example is Culpeper Community Garden, which is open every day of the year and free to all visitors. Plot holders pay a nominal yearly fee, but it's also possible to contribute as a volunteer.

Even in highly urbanized and crowded Japan, there are possibilities for urban gardening. The East Japan Railway Company came up with a clever idea. They transformed the rooftops on its train stations into community gardens. Given the little space in many Japanese cities, the plots aren't cheap. Fortunately, anyone can visit them and help those plot holders who need some assistance.

If you have a little bit more time, consider becoming a volunteer at an organic farm that is a part of World Wide Opportunities on Organic Farms (WWOOF). Members of this network offer the opportunity to help at their farms in exchange for food and lodging. Preferred length of visit varies from a few days to a few weeks, but some farmers are open to weekend stays, too.

If no such opportunities exist where you live, you can also grow food at home. You can do it on the balcony, terrace, in your backyard, or even indoors if you don't have much space. Culinary herbs are the easiest to grow indoors. Onions, garlic, potatoes, tomatoes, salad leaves, peppers, and chilies will grow just about anywhere (yes, even on a windowsill). Of course, this isn't the same thing as being out in nature, but the simple act of caring for plants and then enjoying the fruits of your labor will bring you a little closer to nature, too. I used to grow strawberries on my balcony (now I head to my parents' garden for my fix) and as cliché as it sounds, they did taste better than those you can buy in a store or even at a farmer's market.

CHAPTER 22

The Art of Using Our Senses: Touch the World

❧

The last of the five basic senses we'll cover as we discuss ways to interact with the natural world is touch. As with other senses, the best way to boost your enjoyment of nature is to use this sense in a meditative-like manner. Pick a tree or plant that isn't poisonous (urban parks usually don't present such risk; be careful in a less managed natural environment) and feel its texture. Is it hard or soft? Smooth or rough? Can you tell the difference between the leaves of two different plants based on touch alone? One fun exercise is to close your eyes and ask a friend to lead you to a random tree. Feel its bark. Try to imagine how its texture looks and what species it might be. Then ask your friend to lead you away from the tree. Now open your eyes and try to guess which tree you touched.

Don't be afraid to have fun as you're exploring natural surroundings. When I'm on a walk in a forest, I like to pick up the largest pinecones I can find. When I'm by the ocean, I sometimes look for shells or pick up interesting rocks or pieces of washed ashore dead reef. Skipping stones and watching the ripples is another fun touch-based activity enjoyed by people of all ages. Brush your fingers against the grass when you're having a picnic in a local park. Lightly touch the petals of flowers and smell them. If you're out on a hike, use your hands for extra stability and to feel the trail with your fingers, too. Dig in sand at the beach. If you're confident in your swimming abilities, swim in some unchlorinated water—a lake, sea, ocean, or a slow-moving river. To stay safe, choose beaches patrolled by lifeguards. Use a tow float. Always make sure there are no dangerous currents, incoming big swells, marine life, and/or other perils. Alternatively, take a dip in a stream or any other safe wild body of water.

As a safety precaution when trying to feel the nature with your hands, don't reach where you can't see. You don't want to bond with nature through a snake's venom in your blood. Don't touch any wildlife, either. As cute as they might be, wild animals don't enjoy being pet, and many will attack. If they let you touch them, it's probably because they're sick. Even if they aren't, wild animals don't feel comfortable when touched by humans. As a side note, any tourist attraction that claims to be an animal sanctuary and lets visitors touch animals that live there is unscrupulous.

Going barefoot adds yet another dimension to the experience of interacting with nature. Our ancestors walked barefoot all the time. Modern shoes are a recent development. While offering undeniable benefits when it comes to safety and hygiene when walking down dirty city streets, they also carry negative health implications. A study on 180 individuals from three different population groups (Sotho, Zulu, and European) compared their feet to one another's as well as to the feet of 2,000-year-old skeletons. The findings show that people had healthier feet before the invention of shoes. As for modern humans, the often-barefoot Zulu people had the healthiest feet. Meanwhile, habitual shoe-wearers of Europe had the unhealthiest.[145] According to one of the lead researchers of the study, Dr. Bernhard Zipfel, "most of the commercially available footwear is not good for the feet."[146] Main problems come from the inability to achieve a natural gait, increased stress on the ankles and knees, and lower flexibility and mobility of the foot.

Okay, let me stop here before you run away fearing I'll tell you to throw away every pair of shoes you have. If it isn't obvious yet, I'm a devoted barefoot believer, but I won't offer such extreme suggestions. Instead, let me advocate for occasionally exposing your feet to the natural environment—without shoes, without sandals, without flip-flops. Just you and your bare feet on a natural surface.

There's a lot we're missing by putting a physical barrier between our soles and the ground beneath our feet. Of course, shoes have their place and time, but so does walking barefoot. Walking on grass in shoes doesn't offer the same exhilaration as feeling the stalks between your toes. Jogging on a beach barefoot is worlds apart from engaging in the same activity while running down a promenade. This is both sensory-wise as well as when it comes to the workout you're getting through all the additional muscles and tendons you need to use. Easy hiking trails can turn into fascinating adventures as you experience the various textures of the ground beneath your bare soles.

Of course, don't forget about safety precautions, but don't let it deter you from feeling the world with your feet, too. If you're worried about being barefoot in a wild environment, some cities have so-called barefoot parks where you can safely take off your shoes and experience various natural textures under your feet. Such parks are most common in European countries: Germany, Austria, the Netherland, Denmark, France, Hungary, and the United Kingdom. In Asia, one notable example is Seoul in South Korea with more than 150 barefoot parks throughout the city.

There's a lot to digest and a lot of ideas to try when it comes to experiencing nature using all your senses. To make it easier, pick one sense for each natural outing and ignore the rest as you learn how to see more, hear better, discern smells or flavors, or feel different textures. Strive to experience nature in a wide variety of ways so that even a small urban park can bring you the joy of connecting with life that's all around us.

CHAPTER 23

Other Senses Evoked in Nature

ક્જ

Beyond the five basic senses, humans have a variety of other senses. This includes at least five more senses that we can perceive in our daily lives: balance, temperature, pain, sexual stimulation, and proprioception, the sense of self-movement and body position. There's also one we can train: echolocation, or the ability to detect objects by sensing echoes from them. We also have a host of internal senses known as interoceptions, including hunger, thirst, fullness, the activity of the heart, and many more. Out of the five extra senses we can perceive daily, we can easily employ three of them during our natural outings.

The first one is balance. As we strive to use our senses in nature, the aim is often to enjoy yourself. You spot birds hidden among the branches. You listen to various sounds and recognize their source. You touch interesting textures. Balance isn't any different. The best way to use it is through having fun. As you're on a walk in nature, try to find objects on which you can balance. A fallen tree, a small rock, or a steep hiking trail (but definitely not the edge of a cliff) can all be useful to connect with nature using the sense of balance.

Temporarily replacing your inner adult with an inner child can provide an enjoyable experience. Nobody is above the enjoyment derived from doing something goofy in a natural environment. Any sport and activity that requires balance such as surfing, rock climbing, or stand-up paddleboarding is also a good option to immerse in a natural environment.

Movement in general is one of the ways in which we connect with our roots, too. The more playful and wild in its nature it is, the better for our physical and mental health. Shoot for enjoyable varied outdoor activities over repetitive indoor exercises. Choose multi-dimensional sports that train the entire body over an artificial machine-based movement. Pursue flow and grace to be more focused on the present moment. There are various schools of natural movement skills that will teach you how to do so. One example is MovNat, a fitness philosophy teaching natural, useful, adaptive movements. They improve both strength and mobility while at the same time helping connect with the natural environment. Another school espousing similar values is Animal Flow. It's a ground-based movement program designed to improve the function and communication of the "Human Animal", as its founder Mike Fitch calls it.[147]

The second sense is the sense of temperature. As we spend most of the time in our air-conditioned homes, we rarely get to experience something that was an everyday occurrence for our ancestors: fluctuating temperatures. We can only be grateful that in our modern world it's so easy to enjoy thermal comfort. But at the same time, as we live in our comfortable cocoons, we lose a sense of connection with nature and the elements. Temporarily exposing ourselves to various temperatures characteristic of where we live can bring us closer to the natural world, whether it be through freezing cold or stifling heat. Safety disclaimer first: consult your doctor before you do anything extreme.

If you live in a cold climate, one interesting option is winter swimming, or the practice of immersing yourself in a cold body of water for a few minutes. Proponents of this activity (yours truly included) subject themselves to this torture not because they're masochists, but because it improves their mood. Research suggests that winter swimming may indeed improve general well-being.[148] It may also improve antioxidant protection, making winter swimmers less susceptible to upper respiratory tract infections.[149] Winter swimming lets me partake in one of my favorite outdoor activities when the only option for swimmers is an indoor swimming pool. The endorphin rush I get during my session also makes me more aware of the present moment and the immediate surroundings (I swim in my favorite lake).

Those who live in warmer climates might not be able to engage in proper cold-water swimming. They can still opt to swim in water that might not be entirely comfortable, though. If it's warm year-round, there's always an option to periodically—and safely—expose oneself to hot temperatures. It's a good reminder of what used to be normal for our ancestors living without modern technology.

Using the sense of temperature to interact with nature is about forgoing some comfort in exchange for heightened sensations. Frigid wind, cold droplets of rain, or warm sun rays on the bare skin can all make us more attuned to what's around us. These sensations might not always be pleasant, but they're natural to us, and so they can provide a valuable experience.

The last of the additional, easily perceivable senses we can employ in nature is proprioception. Proprioception is the sense of knowing where your body parts are. If you close your eyes, you can still touch your nose—this is the sense of self-movement at work. This is also why we can still walk without losing balance in darkness and why we can even walk without looking at our feet.

Impaired proprioception can lead to balance issues and a lack of coordination. It's easy to observe in those under the influence of alcohol. Any new skill requires proprioception to learn so that we can eventually perform it without using other senses. We wouldn't be able to drive if we had to constantly look at our feet or our hands on the steering wheel. A tennis player wouldn't be able to play if they had to look at their arm while swinging it versus looking where they want to send a ball.

When you walk on a firm surface and then walk on a soft one, your body will also instantly adapt to it without your conscious involvement. Without proprioception, we wouldn't even be able to judge the effort involved in picking up objects. We wouldn't respond to sudden weight changes that cause a reflex to maintain tension in our muscles (it all happens in less than a millisecond).

One of the reasons why spending time indoors is bad for us is because there's little sensory input. For example, running on a treadmill involves less proprioception—and thus is less immersive—than running outdoors on a variety of surfaces. As we explore the outdoors, we improve our spatial awareness with every step. Through being outdoors, and with heightened understanding of our body position in space, we can also feel closer to the natural world. We can feel the resistance of the wind, the various surfaces under our feet, changing scenery, etc. None of this is a factor when engaging in the same activity indoors.

This goes beyond running. Any outdoor activity that involves input to our muscles and joints improves our proprioception. Examples include jumping, pushing, pulling. Activities that involve balance, coordination, or stability like yoga, slacklining, climbing, and throwing or catching balls are best for improving proprioception.

As we talk about other senses evoked in nature, we can't forget about awe, which isn't defined by scientists as a sense, but as an emotion. Nonetheless, it fits the premise of this chapter, too. Positive psychologist Raul Pearsall describes awe in his book *Awe: The Delights and Dangers of Our Eleventh Emotion* as "overwhelming and bewildering sense of connection with a startling universe that is usually far beyond the narrow band of our consciousness." Albert Einstein considered awe a vital human experience: "The most beautiful emotion we can experience is the mysterious. It is the power of all true art and science. He to whom this emotion is a stranger, who can no longer pause to wonder and stand rapt in awe, is as good as dead."[150]

Anything of great beauty, like nature, art, architecture, or music can make us feel awe. The destructive power of a lightning strike or an atomic bomb can also evoke this emotion. So can anything we consider miraculous or more powerful than us, including the cosmos, the vastness of the ocean, the birth of a child, or religion and the supernatural.

Nature as a source of awe is what interests us most here. In a study on the nature of awe (pun intended), participants were asked to think of a natural scene that was beautiful to them. Meanwhile, another group was asked to think of a moment when they felt pride. The nature group was more likely to report a sense of vastness and the disengagement from the self than the pride group. The researchers concluded their findings by saying that awe had "an impact on the content of the self-concept, increasing one's sense of the self as part of a greater whole—a self-concept that de-emphasises the individual self."[151]

Or, to put it in plain words, awe makes us feel insignificant—in a good way—as we ponder something greater than ourselves. As we expose ourselves to awe-inspiring natural environments, we forget about day-to-day concerns and connect with the world around us on a deeper level.

Can we make ourselves feel awe, or is it a fickle emotion we can't control? I daresay we can choose to feel awe—and benefit from its effects—each time we're out in nature. It comes down to letting ourselves ponder the beauty and grandeur of what's around us.

When I'm in a forest, I often remind myself of how old the trees around me are. I think how much they've seen, how much they've withstood. I also think how even the most majestic of them will die one day, replaced by the small saplings now growing in their shadow. I think of all the wildlife, including insects, that are everywhere around me, and how we all form a part of the living world. Lastly, I think of the humbling cycle of life and death that's so visible around us. I look at that flowering tree and that withering one, or that bird soaring up in the sky and its next victim hiding in the grass.

Any experience in nature can produce awe. When I'm surfing, I feel insignificant as I face the raw power of the ocean. When I'm in the mountains, I realize how unimportant my presence on Earth is, which paradoxically provides a certain sense of relief. It's difficult to worry when you get reminded that in the grand scale of things, none of your problems matter.

Awe not only helps us remember that we're a part of something bigger than us but also makes us relinquish control. When I'm surfing, I can't stop a wave that's about to crash on my head. The ocean doesn't care one iota about me. You can only gape at a thunderstorm. There's nothing you can do to stop its destruction. You can only admire the stars in the sky and wonder what it's like out there and why the cosmos even exists. You can't ever hope to understand the secret of it all, other than perhaps after death, which awaits us all: humans, horses, hawks, hamsters, honey bees, and hickory trees alike.

University of Washington psychology professor Peter Kahn has spent much of his career analyzing the relationship humans have with nature. In an interview for Quartz, Kahn says that "Interacting with nature teaches us to live in relation with the other, not in domination over the other: You don't control the birds flying overhead, or the moon rising, or the bear walking where it would like to walk. In my appraisal, one of the overarching problems of the world today is that we see ourselves living in domination over rather than in relation with other people and with the natural world."[152]

I can hardly find a more elegant way to explain this phenomenon and how powerful a teaching experience a sense of awe can be in reminding us to live in relation instead of domination. Let's not forget to evoke this emotion regularly as we explore our beautiful world.

PART 4

Infusing Your Everyday Urban
Life With Nature

Mohammad lives in Muscat, the capital of the Sultanate of Oman, a country with only 0.006 percent of its land forested.[153] Due to the very hot and arid climate, there's very little that can grow in the country. The rugged terrain of the surrounding Hajar Mountains doesn't seem to be hosting much life, either, and hiking there isn't for the unprepared. For most of the year, the heat in the country is so unbearable that only early mornings and late afternoons allow semi-comfortable conditions for daylight outdoor activities.

And yet, Mohammad loves where he lives and doesn't feel like he's detached from nature. He has a few date palms in his backyard, offering some much-needed shade and attracting local birds. In his house, he has natural stone that not only keeps the interior cool, but also makes it beautiful. It has an imperfect, yet perfect at the same time, texture that no artificial material could match. He strives to take a stroll down the beach with his wife at least a couple of times a week to admire the cerulean blue Indian Ocean. On weekends, he packs his family in an off-road pick-up truck. They visit their favorite nearby wadis, valleys with pools or streams of cool water, where they like to take a dip and observe wildlife.

Sammi lives in Hong Kong, a city that could serve as the definition of "urban jungle" with the largest number of skyscrapers of any city in the world. Living in a tiny rental apartment of 170 square feet (16 square meters), there isn't much she can improve in her home to feel closer to nature other than having one plant on a windowsill. Views from her apartment don't offer much nature, either. The only thing she can see from her window are skyscrapers. Three hundred fifty-five buildings with more than 40 floors all around her, to be exact.

And yet, Sammi is a nature lover who gets her fix every day. On her lunch breaks, she heads to Kowloon Park. It's one of her favorite quiet places in the middle of the bustling city, walled on all sides by high-rise buildings. About 100 different wild bird species live in the park. She often carries her camera to take pictures and upload them later on her blog for urban bird watchers. Sammi also participates in message boards for urban nature lovers. She likes sharing her passion for spotting rare birds in the least-expected, most densely populated places. Whenever she has a few hours to spare, she hikes Victoria Peak, the highest hill on Hong Kong island. Home to many species of birds, including the diurnal raptor the black kite, it's her favorite place in the world. Despite living in one of the most urbanized places in the world, it never crossed her mind that she couldn't design her life to be close to nature.

Darryl lives on a farm in North Dakota, with the closest community of Balfour having only 26 inhabitants. To say that nothing happens there would be an understatement. The state tops the lists of the most boring places in America. Without any major tourist attractions, it's the least visited state. It suffers from a stereotype that a more monotonous and devoid-of-life landscape than its hilled countryside of endless fields doesn't exist. All of Darryl's friends have already left, seeking a more exciting life in a big city.

But Darryl is happy where he is. He might not live close to a scenic national park or anywhere close to large, forested areas—it's almost all farmland in the region—but he doesn't suffer from nature-deficit disorder. Passionate about fruit trees, he planted cultivars of apples, plums, cherry, and pears, all carefully selected for the local climate. He loves caring for the trees throughout the seasons, tasting the fruits of his labor, and selling them to locals.

As a proud resident of North Dakota, the number-one honey-producing state in the nation, he also keeps bees. It's a hobby to connect with nature and a way to generate some side income. Darryl likes to give some honey to his urban-living friends and family and educate them about his passion. He also shares his experience with other beekeepers across the country on a message board for apiculturists. Despite being surrounded by farmland in all directions, Darryl has found a way to connect with nature on his own terms.

These fictional examples show that regardless of where we live, we make the choice of how much nature surrounds us. While in some places this might be trickier than in others, a willing person can still design their life to be rich in various encounters with other life forms. Through embracing technology, biophilic interior design, and taking on a role of an environmental steward, our everyday urban lives can be still infused with nature.

CHAPTER 24

Can Technology and Nature Coexist?

ֶ

In our modern, urbanized world struggling with environmental issues, technology is sometimes painted as the worst enemy. We've already explored that human progress often sadly comes at a cost of the environment. Despite that, it doesn't mean technology has no use for those who want to connect with nature. In fact, quite the contrary. It can help us bond with life and even help us protect it.

For example, thanks to blockchain technology, it's now possible to track the origin of agricultural commodities and fish. This helps stamp out illegal fishing and avoid supporting companies that don't adhere to sustainability practices. Remote sensors, drones, thermal-imaging video cameras, and crowdsourcing help monitor illegal logging and poaching. Camera traps combined with artificial intelligence help collect thousands of photos of wildlife and aid in conservation efforts. And these are just a few examples that portray how beneficial technology can be for protecting the environment.

But how do we approach technology on an individual level? As average people, how can we use it in a way that will help us bond with nature?

The Greatest Danger of Technology

The main challenge of using technology is that it's addictive and distracting. In an article written by Molly Flatt for BBC Earth on the relationship between nature and technology, there's a picture of children relaxing in the countryside.[154] If you imagined them playing in the grass, skipping stones, or climbing trees, I'm sad to tell you that you're old-fashioned. The picture shows four kids sitting on a picnic table, each hunched over their favorite device. If you didn't get the memo, this is the next generation in nature.

Of course, the picture is supposed to be a joke, but as they say, many a true word is spoken in jest. Sadly, such behaviors are more and more common in new generations that are more and more detached from the natural world. Professor Peter Kahn, who we met in the chapter on other senses, coined the term "environmental generational amnesia" to describe the disturbing idea that each generation perceives the environment into which it's born, no matter how developed, urbanized or polluted, as the norm. As Kahn wrote in a paper co-authored with doctoral student Thea Weiss, "With each ensuing generation, the amount of environmental degradation increases, but each generation tends to perceive that degraded condition as the nondegraded condition, as the normal experience."[155]

For a handy metaphor, imagine that you're born in a normal world with all the colors of a rainbow. Then a strange thing happens, and the red color goes missing. You notice it immediately, and the world is no longer the same for you. Your children are born in a world with one of the colors missing, but since that's how the world has always appeared to them, they consider it normal. Then another color, blue, goes missing, too. Your children miss it, and you now miss two colors. But their children—your grandchildren—consider the world without the blue color or the red color normal. Generation by generation, as the phenomenon keeps repeating and stealing away colors, standards get lower and lower until everyone accepts that the world is black and white.

Sadly, this is happening all over the world as children grow up in cities, glued to their devices. They don't get enough natural exposure, often because their parents are overprotective or don't know any better. Some kids develop curiosity and seek to connect with nature themselves. Others fall victim to the distractions presented by technology—social media, video games, etc.—and never gain the skills to interact with the natural environment safely and with respect.

For example, in a Seattle-based preschool, Fiddleheads Forest School, children are taught skills that old-fashioned adults take for granted: mimicking bird calls; digging in the dirt; and, what I found the saddest, even protecting one's body during a fall. As Kahn observed, "We have an entire generation that spends so much time in front of screens that, when they do go out into nature, they don't know how to interact with it, or handle themselves."[156]

I talk about children, but adults—particularly those who grew up in big cities—are also susceptible to this problem. For them, the challenge can be even bigger. They might find it impossible to put down their smartphones, silence them, and immerse themselves in natural surroundings. Even those who love nature often fall victim to the allures of technology (raise your hand if you've never checked your phone while on a nature outing).

This is the bad side of technology we need to be aware of. Just as sometimes in nature there's a poisonous plant growing in the same area as its antidote, so too are there solutions co-existing nearby the way we currently live. In the case of technology, we can remedy its poisonous, distracting nature by using it to arouse curiosity. We can also use it to increase understanding, inspire us to get outdoors, or (paradoxically, given its distracting nature) remind us to stay mindful. Let's explore a few simple and free tools that can help us accomplish those aims.

Simple Tools for Nature Lovers

As we've already explored in the chapter on awareness, education helps us appreciate nature and inspires us to learn more about it. This is a good starting point to begin using technology in a way that will reinforce our relationship with nature. This brings me to one of my favorite tools: Google Maps. I know, I know, it doesn't sound glamorous if you expected a secret app for nature lovers. But hear me out. Google Maps has several useful functions for nature lovers.

The first one is using it to identify the green areas in the region (green spaces are marked with light green color on the map). I routinely look at the map of my area or wherever I find myself in the world for some inspiration on where to go. I use it both to identify wild areas nearby I haven't visited yet as well as possible quiet green places in more urbanized areas. Scouting for potential places to interact with nature keeps things interesting. Instead of visiting the same places over and over again, you can keep exploring your city and its surroundings even if you've lived there your entire life. I take great pleasure in getting to know my area and its lesser known natural attractions. I later share them with my friends. It's an extra reward, and you get the benefits of nature exposure to boot.

Another useful function of Google Maps is Street View. It provides interactive panoramas not only of streets, but also of rural areas and sometimes even wild areas, including hiking trails, landscape views, and more. Finding a green area on the map is a good first step. If you can also virtually immerse yourself in it through using Street View, you can get a rough idea of what it's like and whether you'll enjoy it.

The interactive panoramas come from Google as well as from contributors. This brings me to the third point: you too can contribute by taking 360-degree photos or regular photos and uploading them on Google Maps. This way, technology can not only help you explore new places but will also make your interactions more rewarding through sharing the experience with others.

Google Lens is another great aid for those who want to deepen their understanding of nature. Available as a mobile app, it provides image recognition and brings up relevant information related to the portrayed object. For example, you can take a picture of a leaf and learn to what tree species it belongs. The app can also recognize various plants, flowers, and animals, being your handy personal wilderness expert. Google Lens doesn't always recognize the objects properly, particularly if it's a non-descript tiny leaf of a shrub. So, if you still need help identifying something in nature, you can turn to other plant-identifying apps. Type "identify plants" in the app store of your device for the current best options. If the apps that rely on machine learning don't help, turn to community-based apps, where plant experts will help you identify a given plant, flower, or tree. A quick search of available apps will also reveal that there are apps to help identify animal tracks and bird song. I'm not recommending anything in particular. The apps come and go. By the time you read this, there might be new apps, so it's best to test what's currently available yourself.

Moving on from the educating role of technology, let's now cover mindfulness. It sounds unlikely that technology can help us develop more self-awareness, given how much it steals our attention, yet it can—if we use the right apps. For example, if you're struggling to calm your mind as you're out in nature, you can let a meditation app like Headspace or Calm guide you through the practice. I prefer not to use technology while meditating, but whether you use an app or not, a few minutes of quiet focus as you sit by a tree or on the beach can heighten the sensations you feel in nature. Meditation is also easier outdoors. If you don't believe me, a study by researchers at the Uppsala University in Sweden suggests that a natural meditation setting helps people stick to mindfulness training.[157]

Let's move on to the third category of tools that help bond with nature: those that help by making our natural outings easier or that help record our trips. One of my favorite tools is Strava, an app that lets you track your physical activity, including drawing on a map in real time your trail, duration, and pace. For some reason, using the app makes it even more fun to get outdoors—perhaps it's the data geek in me that loves to track my activity.

Originally created for cyclists and runners, Strava now offers tracking of other activities, too. It can track walking, hiking, canoeing, skiing, swimming, stand-up paddling, and more. When I'm swimming outdoors, I put my phone in a waterproof bag in my tow float and let Strava record my workout. Later I can check my stats and the route I took (unfortunately, sometimes the GPS signal gets lost and routes aren't recorded properly). I love swimming, but with recorded data I enjoy it even more.

You can use the app for any of your favorite activities, for example to keep record of your hiking trails and to share them with others. A popular alternative to Strava is Endomondo. Unfortunately, I found that Endomondo often had issues. Many times it failed to record the activity, which is why I switched to more reliable Strava.

As for hiking, great tools that can help plan your trips are AllTrails and WikiLoc. These websites consist of giant databases of hiking trails all over the world. Both are available as a mobile app, too. If you're unsure where to go in your area, type your location on the website or in the app to discover new trails. Trails come not only with basic information like length, difficulty, pictures, directions on the map and elevation profile. They also come with valuable tips and reviews of fellow hikers including how crowded and difficult it was. Note that you don't have to be a hiker or live in a town surrounded by wilderness to benefit from AllTrails and WikiLoc. The database also offers walking trails, running trails, and biking trails in urban areas. If your area is not available or features few trails, a quick Google search is all you need to find other opportunities. You can also use social media to find local hiking groups and join them on a group hike.

Another technological aid I use is a service called where2go provided by weather forecast website meteoblue.com. This function shows you where you can expect the best weather near a chosen area. It takes into account longer sunshine hours and lower precipitation probability.

Why is this better than a simple forecast?

It's because where2go shows you exactly which specific nearby area will get best weather in the morning, afternoon, the entire day, or up to four days ahead. This might be a little dot on the map for which the software predicts best conditions. You can choose from a radius between 30 to 500 kilometers of your chosen location (it's a European website working globally; in miles, it's approximately 19 to 311 miles).

I mostly use the first two ranges—30 kilometers and 60 kilometers (19 miles and 38 miles). The first range is useful if you don't have time for longer trips and want to identify the part of the city or its nearest surroundings that will get the best weather. For example, if you're not sure which park to choose, see which area will get better weather and go there. Exploring nature in pleasant conditions is more enjoyable than enduring bad weather. You want to immerse yourself in nature, not hope to get home as soon as possible because you're cold or dripping wet.

I find this tool useful year-round. When it's winter and I'm sun deprived, I choose where to go for a walk or for a day trip depending on what where2go suggests. Sometimes merely driving 20 minutes in one direction rather than going in the other makes the difference between partly sunny weather and cloudy skies. In the summer or on vacation, I often use this tool to decide where to go hiking or which nearby natural attractions to visit.

For example, I once went with some friends on a trip to Bieszczady Mountains. As any other mountain range, the weather there can be fickle. The forecast wasn't particularly promising when we arrived. In addition to cloudy weather, it predicted thunderstorms that precluded any hiking. Fortunately, where2go came to the rescue. It identified which specific areas would get the best weather. We chose hiking trails in those zones. Thanks to this tool, we avoided rain and even enjoyed sunny weather and some beautiful views of the green polonynas (a specific geographic name for montane meadows in the Carpathians). Meanwhile, there were thunderstorms in other areas. Yes, my friends were impressed with my magical forecasting skills, but I owe all the credit to meteoblue.com.

Of course, the tool isn't always perfect. If you're going anywhere where adverse weather conditions can be dangerous (i.e. mountains or other wilderness areas), be cautious. Still, where2go is one of my favorite technological aids to make sure that as I enjoy natural surroundings, I also enjoy the best weather possible.

Virtually Immersing Ourselves in Nature

Thanks to modern technology, if you can't interact with nature in the physical world, you can still get some benefits. Research suggests that there may be a benefit in viewing nature pictures and videos (also defined by scientists as "simulated natural environment") through improving attention[158] and reducing stress.[159]

One of the tools for simulating natural environments we've already explored is Google Street View and its panoramic 360-degree photos. The tool isn't only useful for urban and near-urban areas. You can also use it to explore some of the world's most awe-inspiring destinations. For example, you can take a virtual journey down the Colorado River. You can explore the remote Khumbu Valley in the shadow of Mt. Everest. You can visit the Samburu National Reserve in Kenya. It's even possible to virtually dive in the Great Barrier Reef, or climb El Capitan in Yosemite National Park.

Will it be the same as the actual experience? Of course not. Real natural exposure, even if it's a brief walk in a local urban park, is better than watching interactive panoramas of exotic destinations. It employs more senses and you're actually *there*. But if you don't have other options, Street View is still better than nothing, particularly due to its immersive 360-degree quality.

Regular photos and videos have their place, too. Granted, they don't transport you to a given destination in as interactive a way as Street View. Yet they can still provide a sense of awe and appreciation of the natural world. I'm a huge fan of documentaries narrated by David Attenborough. Even if I might never visit some of the places shown in the movies, I can still develop at least a basic understanding of what they're like. I can see what kind of animals populate them, what plants grow there and what natural phenomena is associated with them. Non-interactive photographs can also get us a little closer to nature and inspire us to head outdoors and spot wildlife ourselves. Following blogs or vlogs of nature lovers around the world is another great way to learn more about our beautiful planet. You can get inspired for future travels, gain appreciation of what's around us, or enjoy a quick nature fix if you can't leave your house at the moment.

As we've already explored, curiosity and education spark the need to engage with the natural world. Any digital natural experience can be helpful if it encourages us to create your own real-world experiences in the actual, physical world.

What Technology Can't Do

No matter how immersive virtual reality devices become or how engaging and crisp nature documentaries get, they can never replace the actual, real exposure to nature. We might use these tools for inspiration or as an alternative when we can't experience nature ourselves. Stuck in a cubicle, it's better to look at images of nature during a lunch break than waste time on social media. But we can't ever forget that in the end we humans, as much as we love technology, come from the natural environment. We might be able to teleport ourselves to natural worlds through video games, virtual reality, or videos. But even with a growing number of senses these technological inventions can elicit, they lack two key features of nature that can't and won't be imitated.

One of them is immediate, palpable consequences of our actions. A video game might expose us to difficult situations and punish us for wrong choices. However, it doesn't invoke the sense of exposure and survival that nature provides in spades, immediately and often painfully. For example, if you play a climbing video game and you fall, you just restart the game. In the real world, the stakes are higher, and so the experience is more immersive as it requires you to prepare and be more attuned to the world around you. That's not to say I encourage participating in risky activities or being ignorant of the dangers of the wilderness. Outdoor climbing can be relatively safe as long as you adhere to safety precautions. But while it will never be as safe as playing a video game, a virtual world will never provide the abundance of deep sensory experiences of the physical world.

In the same way, you might see beautiful shots of the ocean or even swim in one with a virtual reality set, but you'll never get to experience the warmth (or the cold) of the water. You won't feel the breeze and the sunrays on your skin. You won't experience a little sense of danger or exposure that comes from immersing in a natural environment. There's a risk-reward balance we need to find here, but isn't that variety of emotion and the feeling of being alive what we also seek in nature?

The second feature of spending time in actual nature is that the physical world provides a sense of freedom and a certain lack of control. Virtual environments and videos are manufactured things. Limited in their nature, they only allow you to see and experience what the creator of the game or the film director provides. As for control, you can always turn off a game or fast-forward a video if you don't like a particular moment or feel bored.

Out in nature, any encounter you have is unmoderated. It lies largely outside your control, unscripted and random. Unfortunately, you can't remove yourself from a hiking trail if it turns out to be too challenging. At the same time, you can't predict when you'll see a majestic manifestation of nature, whether it's a herd of wild animals, a natural phenomenon, or a beautiful landscape. Again, with freedom and a lack of control comes the risk, but what may also follow is a rich experience and inspiring adventures.

When Is Technology Helpful? The Final Answer

There's one simple filter we can use to judge whether a piece of technology can help us get closer to nature. Did it inspire real-world action that made us head to a natural environment or provide emotions we experience in nature?

You might not be heading to the exotic destinations you saw in a BBC documentary. However, if the film inspired you to go and explore your local surroundings, it was still helpful. If listening to recordings of birds or going on a virtual tour of a natural landmark has improved your mood, then technology, indirectly, has also helped you bond with nature.

Or let's consider a thirteen-year old playing a video game featuring natural landscapes. If it only makes them interested in scoring more points in the virtual environment, as opposed to actually *caring* about the natural environment, its usefulness in inspiring a deeper connection with non-virtual life is debatable.

If a person heads outdoors only to take a few selfies, ignorant and uninterested in the world around them, then that particular area of technology also poses a barrier to bonding with nature.

Technology can lead teenagers to addictive hobbies. It can glue them to their screens and make them spend entire days indoors. But at the same time it can also help us design more nature-friendly homes and infuse them with life. Thanks to countless scientific advancements, everyone can bring some nature indoors. This is what we're going to explore in the next chapter.

CHAPTER 25

Designing a Nature-Friendly Home

ఎ

Since we spend most of the time in our homes, it makes sense to turn them into nature-friendly oases, doesn't it? This way, even if we can't spend much time outside interacting with natural landscapes, we can still enjoy small daily doses. In this chapter we'll discuss some ways to accomplish this goal. We'll do so by following the principles of "biophilic design." It's a concept used within the building and interior design industries that aims to increase the occupant's connection with nature. Let's start with the first, most obvious step to make your home more nature friendly.

Indoor Plants to the Rescue

Houseplants have a long history, with the earliest written evidence of their use dating back to the Egyptians in the third century BC.[160] For most of the next two thousand-plus years, indoor plants were mostly reserved for the wealthy. Orangeries were a prime example of indoor nature reserved for the well-off. They were popular among noblemen and rich merchants between the 17th and 19th centuries. Then the world urbanized. It was cheaper and easier to grow and transport subtropical and tropical plants around the globe. As a result, more people, and not just the rich, could afford to keep houseplants.

Today, an average city dweller, on an average day, might see more indoor plants than outdoor plants. They're a must-have element of interior design of trendy offices, glitzy shopping malls, high-end restaurants, hotels, waiting areas, and of course, our homes. Thanks to modern HVAC systems, there are no geographic bounds. Everyone around the world can enjoy subtropical and tropical plants indoors.

As we've already mentioned in the chapter on indoor pollution, houseplants aren't effective at improving indoor air quality. They may only work if you manage to fit between 10 and 1,000 plants per 10 square feet (one square meter) into your space. The range is so wide because even scientists aren't sure about the plants' properties.[161] Plants might not help filter air even a tenth as effectively as airing out your house.

However, they serve another important function that does have a noticeable impact on our lives. A meta-analysis of various experimental studies suggests that indoor plants may offer psychological benefits. This includes reduced stress and increased pain tolerance.[162] Note the word "suggests." Given few quality studies and the difficulty of studying the subject, we can't say with absolute conviction if, and how, houseplants, affect our well-being. But do we need studies to convince us to bring a little nature into our homes and see how it impacts us?

There's no need to seek expensive, exotic plants or have a green thumb. Common houseplants you can buy in any garden center are affordable, easy to care for, and beautiful to look at. I'm particularly fond of peace lilies (*Spathiphyllum*). They tolerate a variety of light conditions, with medium to bright spots preferable. They grow quickly, have big, beautiful leaves, and produce pretty white flowers year-round.

Swiss cheese plant (*Monstera deliciosa*) is another fast-growing plant. It has big leaves and adds a lot of greenery with little maintenance needed.

Lucky bamboo (*Dracaena sanderiana*) is another common plant that tolerates even the least-talented gardeners. It has twisted bamboo-like stems and long, narrow leaves. You don't even need a pot to grow it. It's happy even in a vase filled with water.

Another hardy plant is yucca. Place it in a sunny spot, water it sparingly, and it will grow quickly, injecting a little bit of a desert-feel in your interior design.

If you need a plant that tolerates low light, low humidity, and drought, ZZ plant (*Zamioculcas zamiifolia*) with its waxy smooth leaves is a perfect choice.

Mother-in-law's Tongue, or the snake plant (*Dracaena trifasciata*), can survive even up to a month of neglect.

Finally, if you want an easy to grow fast-growing vine, pothos or the devil's ivy (*Epipremnum aureum*) is what you want.

You can see how some of these plants look by checking extra resources on my website at *www.MartinSummerAuthor.com*. The password to access bonus resources is "connecting."

If you can't or don't want to have houseplants, fresh flowers can introduce a little nature in your home, too. Choose flowers that have the longest lifespan—zinnias, orchids, or carnations—which can all last up to three weeks. To make fresh flowers last longer, change their water every other day. Remove dead leaves and petals that fall into the water. Keep them in a cool room. Adding some baking soda to a vase is a simple trick to make the blooms last longer, too.

A more recent trend is to install so-called "green walls"—waterproof systems you mount on a wall that allow vertical gardening indoors. They can be made of the same common plants kept indoors or of dormant moss that requires little to no maintenance (not even watering). If you go for the latter, make sure that the moss was preserved using environmentally friendly, biodegradable preservative. Done properly, a moss wall will keep its natural appearance and vivid green color for at least a decade. If you want to make your house greener without adding another chore to your list, this might be a great investment.

One caveat is that indoor plants may promote mold growth and be potential allergy triggers. To eliminate mold from houseplants, wipe off the leaves with a moist paper towel or give them a shower, which will also help get rid of dust and dirt. In more extreme cases, using a fungicide (preferably a natural one such as tea tree oil, jojoba oil, oregano oil, or baking soda) might be in order. Overwatering plants contributes to mold growth, and so does keeping them in dark places with low air circulation.

Gardening

If you're blessed to have a backyard where you can cultivate plants, you can bring wild nature right onto your doorstep. I won't pretend to be a great gardener. Because I currently live in an apartment, I have limited experience with gardening. I planted a small native forest in my parents' backyard following the Miyawaki method (I highly suggest learning more through free resources at *www.afforestt.com*). I also help them cultivate some vegetables and fruits. I'm not a fan of manicured, obviously man-made gardens so my experience caring for them is non-existent. I favor wild landscapes (and backyards) of life-attracting native species.

Native plants attract local insects, which in turn attract local birds that feast on them. Exotic, ornamental species, or worst of all from the perspective of biodiversity, lawns, provide none of the benefits. Moreover, native species are easier to cultivate as they're adapted to the local conditions. They don't need fertilizers or pesticides (or they need less of them). They need less water, which is particularly important in dry climates where xeriscaping is preferential to water-consuming lawns. They often grow faster. They promote natural landscapes and heritage. A great book that goes into more detail about the importance of growing native plants is *Bringing Nature Home* by Douglas W. Tallamy.

Growing fruits and vegetables, particularly those cultivated in your region for thousands of years, is also a great way to bring nature close to you. You'll also gain a valuable experience of caring for the plants and tasting the fruits (and vegetables) of your labor. As we've already discussed, even if you don't have much space, you can still grow some fruits, vegetables, and herbs indoors. So, if you live in a small apartment, don't use that as an excuse that you can't be a gardener! Even growing parsley on a kitchen windowsill alone can be a fun, low-effort hobby and a way to bring some nature indoors (that's what I do).

Natural Light

We've already explored how important natural light is for our well-being. Given how little natural light we get as we spend the majority of our days hunched over our desks or smartphones, we should strive to bring more natural light indoors. It will lift our spirits, give us more energy, and increase our property values. Let's explore a few easy fixes to brighten up our homes.

The first easy trick to increase natural light is to focus on reflecting light throughout the room. Light colors on walls make a space feel brighter. They reflect the natural light entering the room instead of absorbing it like dark colors. Off-white shades are best. They increase the amount of natural light and avoid the cold feel of brilliant white. Paint the ceiling a few shades lighter than the walls to make the space appear taller, larger, and brighter. The best type of paint for reflecting light is gloss, then semi-gloss, and lastly satin. However, the shinier the paint, the more any imperfections will stand out, so you need to choose between aesthetics and more light.

Highly reflective tiles in bathrooms and kitchens will make them bigger and brighter, too. Furniture and accessories with a reflective surface such as metallic, chrome, or glass will also reflect light, making the space brighter and bigger. Conversely, dark furniture and accessories absorb light. Putting a mirror across from a window or on the wall next to it is another easy fix that may double the amount of light that enters the room. If you're renting, it's the most effective fix that won't put you at odds with your landlord.

Another quick fix is to move any furniture and accessories that block light from windows. Moving a bookshelf or a sofa that's by a window will immediately increase the amount of light. It will also give you more opportunities to increase it even further through reflection. Don't forget about shades, curtains, drapes, and blinds. They might be helpful to avoid artificial light at night, but they take up a lot of light during the day. Pull them up or to the side (unless you have nosy neighbors or your house heats up too much).

Flooring can also make a huge difference to the amount of natural light, although it's a more expensive solution than the previously discussed fixes. Carpets can make a room feel warmer, but they don't reflect much light (if you love carpets, choose light colors). Wooden floors (particularly natural wood due to additional reasons we'll discuss later) are a better choice. If you live in a warm climate, ceramic or stone floors will not only brighten the space but also make it cooler.

Another more expensive but effective solution is installing new, larger windows. One of the best improvements I've done to my apartment was tearing down a part of a wall in the bedroom to install glass doors leading onto the balcony. This way, a previously dark room now receives more natural light and has a better view, too. If you live in a house, you can also consider skylights and more affordable and less messy solar tubes.

Don't forget to clean your windows regularly. A lot of dust accumulates on them, particularly if you live in a big city. Keep the greenery you have on your windowsills or outside under control. Plants are great, but if they block natural light, it might be worth it to move them or trim them a little. As much as I love houseplants, I don't keep any on a windowsill in a north-facing room. It gets little daylight, and any plants would make it even darker than it already is.

If you live in a hot climate, you might be more interested in reducing the amount of sunlight entering your home to keep it cool. Even if the biggest asset of a property in your region is the amount of shade, make sure that while you seek to cool down, you don't reduce the amount of natural light to unhealthy levels. Consider cooling off your house through creating a cross-breeze effect. You can also use naturally cool materials. Try to avoid turning your house into a dark air-conditioned cave.

Fresh Air

Stagnant air doesn't feel good, and it most definitely doesn't feel like nature (caves excluded). We explored the dangers of low indoor air quality and some potential fixes in the second part of the book. Strategies include not smoking indoors, minimizing clutter, vacuuming, and using natural cleaning supplies over those with harsh chemicals. To expand on this topic, here are a few more suggestions to enjoy fresh air in your home.

First, focus on natural ventilation, which is a key aspect of a healthy, nature-friendly home. You can't do much without modifying the house which requires professional advice. However, I couldn't skip this topic and ignore mentioning the need for good natural air flow. If you aren't using air conditioning and the outdoor air quality is good, open doors and windows to increase air flow and get rid of the stale air. Early mornings or late evenings are usually best. On warm days, aim to get that nice cross-breeze effect going. Using fans in combination with open windows is even better. Remember to keep vents unblocked and clean, and don't skip on HVAC maintenance. Aim to keep humidity between 30 percent and 50 percent to keep allergens under control.

Dust mites that so much enjoy our bedding, cushions and curtains reduce indoor air quality, too. That's why it's important to regularly wash these items. Carpets and rugs also attract dust. It's best not to use them or vacuum them regularly if you want to maximize the amount of fresh air indoors. Air purifiers can be a sensible investment if ventilating your house and keeping it clean don't help achieve desired air quality.

Prevent contaminants from entering your home by using a large door mat and wiping your shoes. Or better yet, if possible, leave them outside Hawaiian-style. We track a lot of dirt, chemicals, and other pollutants on our shoes. Leave them outside, not on the floors in your home.

If you want your home to smell good without adding dozens of chemicals to the air, stay away from synthetic fragrances and choose natural products. Baking soda can help absorb unpleasant smells. Essential oils in a diffuser will not only bring natural smells indoors, but will also, unlike chemical-laden air fresheners, provide other health benefits associated with aromatherapy.

Water

Bringing water into our living spaces is tricky, but a chapter about biophilic design wouldn't be complete without at least a brief mention of it. If you're blessed to live in a place with a waterfront view, you're covered. If not, one simple way to add some water in your interior design is through a small indoor fountain. The sound of moving water will help drown out unwanted noise. If you have more time and money, consider aquascaping, or underwater gardening. It's a hobby of arranging plants, stones, rocks, and other natural features in aquariums. You don't need fish to create your own underwater landscape. If you want even less maintenance, you can use only rocks, stones, and driftwood.

If you have a backyard, you can put water features in place more easily through fountains or ponds. However, their cost, maintenance, and the increased risk of unwanted visitors like mosquitos might outweigh their benefits.

Natural Materials

A biophilic home strengthens our connection with nature through a variety of senses. We've already covered the main ways to use our sight, hearing, sense of smell, and even taste. Time for touch.

Natural materials are a must-have element in nature-friendly interiors. They offer tactility that most synthetic materials lack. Whether it's wood, bamboo, rattan, wicker, stone, or cotton, they all have a distinct quality due to the variation in their texture. Their imperfect, random nature with all the unique knots, rings, lines, grains, bumps, and spots makes them nuanced and pleasant to the touch. The warm feel and look of a hardwood floor is worlds apart from artificial, synthetic wood. Likewise, sitting in a plastic chair offers little pleasure compared to sitting in a beautifully made rattan or wicker chair.

Another aspect of natural materials that makes them so interesting is that they age. As they age, they change their appearance. We might not like aging ourselves, but we do like to observe the passage of time and weathering of natural materials. One evidence is the extraordinary prices of well-aged furniture like dining tables, chairs, or desks, to name a few. Nature is dynamic, so by using the materials that change over time we can introduce some of that element into our houses.

When talking about natural materials, I'd be remiss if I didn't emphasize the importance of buying materials manufactured with stringent sustainability standards. We don't want to decorate our houses to connect with nature by contributing to deforestation. One might argue there's a certain amount of hypocrisy in being a nature lover and using natural materials like hardwood flooring. However, the synthetic alternatives made of toxic chemicals don't strike me as a better alternative. They harm the environment when manufactured, when used, and when disposed of. Furthermore, you can sand down and refinish hardwood floors many times, allowing them to last a lifetime, if not several lifetimes.

Another option is to find an architectural salvage yard and use reclaimed building materials for your nature-inspired interior design. This way, you'll save money, decorate your house with a distinct aged piece, and reduce your ecological footprint.

Natural Colors

Neutral subdued colors found in nature—browns, greens, and blues characteristic of soil, plants, rocks, the sky, and water—are best for those who want to make their homes more biophilic. Artificial, bright, and contrasting colors are unnatural. They may be distracting or even fatiguing when overdone. When in doubt, stick to earth colors that are neutral and go well with everything. To mimic natural environments and avoid dullness, sprinkle in some brighter colors through flowering houseplants, fresh flowers, colorful pillows with natural patterns, or art. A speck of vivid colors found in nature can break the monotony of a monochromatic room.

Natural Patterns and Shapes

There's a multitude of patterns and shapes that evoke nature. There are leaves, trees, and flowers. There are wings, shells, waves, honeycomb, ripples, symmetry, spirals, meanders, bubbles, cracks, spots, and stripes. Fractals, patterns that repeat themselves as they get smaller or larger, are also common. You can observe them in ferns, corals, clouds, snowflakes, and frost crystals on glass.

All of these forms can transform a dull, static room into a space that feels more alive and pleasant to look at through using natural geometry that attracts the human eye (and particularly that of a nature lover!).

The Imperfections of Nature

Nature is perfect in its imperfection. We like natural landscapes because, unlike uniform man-made landscapes, they're interesting to look at with all the randomness they offer. Straight lines and rectangles abound in our cities, but nature is always a little off. Even when something is almost identical, it's always a little different in size, shape, or texture. Nature can be complex and organized but at the same time it can be chaotic. We can bring some of those features indoors. We can do it through embracing some variety, randomness, and resisting the temptation to make everything perfectly arranged in our homes.

For example, consider plants of different species, with different heights, taking up different amounts of space. They're more aesthetic and invoke nature better than a neat row of trimmed plants of the same height, each in the same boring pot.

Aged furniture or any other natural material that has acquired a patina of time, thus making it look imperfect compared to a shiny new object, will also inject more nature into a room. Instead of buying a new piece of furniture, consider refurbishing what you already have. The effects can be amazing if it's of high-quality and made of natural materials.

In Japanese aesthetics, there's a philosophy called "wabi-sabi" that espouses the acceptance of imperfection, impermanence, and incompletion. The concept is derived from Buddhist teachings, but I can't help but see a striking similarity to biophilic design. In both philosophies, we aim to integrate natural objects and processes into our lives. We accept their transience and imperfect nature. Wabi-sabi is loosely translated as "wisdom in natural simplicity" or "flawed beauty." And what is biophilic design if not a search for the same things through daily connection with nature?

Since wabi-sabi aims to appreciate imperfect authenticity and the beauty of age, items that best represent this philosophy (and make our homes more biophilic) include original pieces made of natural materials. This doesn't mean seeking used, broken furniture or accessories just to have something "imperfect" in your room. Instead, it means not being afraid to display such items if they bring you joy and evoke feelings of connection with nature and its impermanence. I pour tea from an old-fashioned cast iron tea kettle called a *tetsubin* (also a Japanese invention). Iron and water equals rust. No matter what you do, orange discoloration will appear shortly. You may deem it imperfect and ugly, or you can embrace it as a beautiful expression of natural processes.

Another aspect of wabi-sabi is sustainability. Find new, creative or quirky, uses of items that might no longer serve their original purpose. An old woolen sock may serve as a flower pot cover. A coconut shell can be a small bowl. An ugly jumper in a cardboard box can be your cat's favorite warm bed.

Bringing out the new layer of beauty in what we already have (or learning to see it despite imperfections) is not only environmentally friendly. It also helps us accept the passage of time, a quality that we've also discussed in the chapter on the other senses evoked in nature. One notable expression of this, often found in Japanese homes designed with wabi-sabi in mind, are pottery items that look rustic, unrefined, and asymmetric. They sometimes even have cracks or chips in them. The next time your favorite mug or bowl shatters into a manageable amount of pieces, don't be afraid to glue it back together and give it a place of honor that will draw attention.

Images of Nature

Lastly, we have images of nature, providing an indirect but still observable experience of connecting with it. They might not provide the same level of engagement as the other suggestions listed in this chapter. Nonetheless, images are an element of biophilic design. But repeated exposure, versus just a single image, is key. According to the *Practice of Biophilic Design* by Stephen R. Kellert and Elizabeth F. Calabrese, "Single or isolated images of nature typically exert little impact. Representational expressions of nature should be repeated, thematic, and abundant."

There's a variety of decorations you can use to bring visual representations of nature into your spaces. You don't have to rely on wallpapers or framed prints and photographs alone. You can also introduce natural patterns (leaves, flowers, birds, etc.) on your cushions, bedsheets, blankets, tablecloths, curtains, rugs, towels, and other textiles. It can also work on furniture and accessories, including vases, lamps, mirrors, or even your glasses and mugs. You can also consider wall stencils for paintings that represent nature— for example, trees, floral designs, leaves, birds, mountains, or even entire landscapes.

For examples of biophilic interior design, head over to my website at *www.MartinSummerAuthor.com*. I published an article there showing a few dozen examples of bringing nature into your home. Again, the password to access bonus resources is "connecting."

CHAPTER 26

Stewardship Is More Important Than Ever Before

ð.

There's no shortage of horrible stories from around the world about how our planet is changing. Both virgin environments as well as nature in cities are threatened by short-sighted projects that destroy the local environment for a fast injection of cash or new urban developments in areas where land is getting increasingly expensive.

As a child, I used to spend a lot of time on an overgrown, tree- and bush-covered vacant plot of land bordering a forest right by where I lived. It was a wild oasis where my friends and I had great adventures from sunrise to sunset. Several years ago, the plot turned into a big construction site. First, a swimming pool appeared. Then more sports facilities were added—smack dab where we used to climb small hills, pretending to be blacksmiths, knights, or great explorers. The wild land from my childhood is gone. It's replaced by levelled ground and fenced buildings with sparse trees of a dwarf species (for which, I have to admit, I have a particular animosity, given how unnatural they look and how little they offer for local wildlife).

The story of this single plot of land is nothing compared to the vast destruction around the world. To say that urbanization has been tough on the environment would be a grand understatement. More than 77 percent of land (excluding Antarctica) and 87 percent of the ocean has been modified by the direct effects of human activities.[163] Few true wilderness areas without a human footprint remain. Most are located in hard-to-reach destinations. The wild areas an average person might possibly visit—such as popular national parks—unfortunately struggle with some major challenges. These issues spoil our experience of exploring them as well as, more importantly, damage the local environment and cause disruptions to the wildlife.

For example, an article on noise pollution in U.S. protected areas shows that noise generated by humans—including that from transportation, development, and the extraction of natural resources—threatens the survival of plant and animal species across the country. The study offers disturbing findings. Man-made noise doubled background sound levels in 63 percent of U.S. protected areas and caused a 10-fold or greater increase in 21 percent of them.[164] Some parks suffer from air pollution caused by nearby power plants, industry, and vehicles. For example, a whitish haze caused by pollution sometimes obscures views in the Great Smoky Mountains. High levels of ground level ozone in the park can also cause respiratory issues to visitors. They also damage trees and other plants. The park also suffers from acid rain, acid clouds, and nitrogen overload. This, in turn, hurts both vegetation and streams.[165]

To connect with nature and encourage others to do the same, we as individuals also run the risk of overexploiting the natural environments. Each year, nearly 100 million pounds of waste are generated in national parks in the United States.[166] Even remote parks like Denali National Park struggle with waste brought from outside the park. The scale of the problem was particularly visible during the 2019 U.S. government shutdown. The lack of staffing and security resulted in piles of dumped trash, vandalism, and dirty bathrooms. This isn't just aesthetics. Overflowing toilets can cause damage to water and soil. Leftover food can attract wildlife to camping areas, causing potentially dangerous encounters between animals and human visitors.

There's also visitor-caused pollution in less permanent forms that nonetheless detracts from the experience. I'm talking about bright tents, colorful clothing, stacks of stones (Zion National Park calls the practice destructive and says that it's "simply vandalism"[167]), loud conversations, and crowds at the most popular scenic outlooks.

Yet again, we aren't talking merely about aesthetics. Wildlife ecologist Tom Smith investigated the effect of brightly colored tents on bear visitation in

Alaska's Katmai National Park. The park is more densely populated with brown bears (grizzlies) than anywhere else on Earth. He found that bear visitation immediately decreased upon switching to camouflage shelters. It turns out that brown bears are very curious. Any novelty—including garish colors absent in nature—grabs their attention and tempts them to investigate. Black bears aren't different from brown bears. According to black bear biologist Tom Beck, once a black bear spots the specks of color from a distance, it will abandon what it's doing and come to investigate.[168] (If you're concerned about not having a possible emergency signal to see you from the air, use a camouflaged rainfly with a brightly-colored tent.)

Even when not in bear country, do we want to see neon-colored plastic shelters and people donning bright clothes dotting the natural landscape? Do we enjoy hiking to the tune of loud conversations and shutter sounds? Do we want to see natural wonders destroyed by vandals? Do we want to see trampled vegetation, trash, stacks of stones, and other signs of human presence by our favorite trails?

One of my least favorite hiking experiences was in the Krkonoše Mountains in Czechia. Every couple of minutes my friend and I passed rolls of toilet paper and human waste right by a trail. To this day, whenever I think about Czechia, the first thing that comes to my mind is what we saw on this day on the trail. Another example of a beautiful place spoiled by the lack of conservation principles was my and my girlfriend's experience in the Ala Archa National Park in Kyrgyzstan. We saw remains of food and other trash left by inconsiderate visitors found at almost every step. It was right by a pristine river with clean water flowing from a glacier!

If you're unsure how to behave in a natural environment (and this includes both remote wilderness areas as well as urban parks), read up on the Seven Principles of Leave No Trace established by The Leave No Trace Center for Outdoor Ethics and available at lnt.org. The philosophy helps educate people on how to take care of our protected areas. But to save nature everywhere—not just in national parks—we should also think beyond what we do in the wilderness. This brings me to *Beyond Leave No Trace*, seven principles suggested by researchers Gregory Simon and Peter Alagona in their controversial essay "Beyond Leave No Trace." Simon and Alagona believe that leave no trace should start at home.[169] These principles can help us protect the environment, whether we mostly interact with nature in our cities or in more remote areas. They are:

1. Educate yourself and others about the places you visit.
2. Purchase only the equipment and clothing you need.
3. Take care of the equipment and clothing you have.
4. Make conscientious food, equipment, and clothing consumption choices.
5. Minimize waste production.
6. Reduce energy consumption.
7. Get involved by conserving and restoring the places you visit.

We don't have to discuss why reducing energy consumption is so important for our environment. However, other principles might need some explaining to better understand the idea behind them.

Simon and Alagona start their list of *Beyond Leave No Trace* principles with educating yourself and others about the places you visit. They emphasize in their essay that we tend to disregard the fact that wilderness areas have changed over time through complex human-environment interactions. Following camping etiquette alone might not be enough to protect them. Learning about the history, geography, and ecology of the places we visit will help us understand the complex challenges they face. This includes, among others, climate change, air pollution, and invasive species (remember the example of Nā Pali Coast State Park). Armed with this knowledge, we can better follow the seventh principle: getting involved by conserving and restoring the places we visit.

Principles two through five come down to the original leave no trace philosophy's failure to address what happens outside of the wilderness areas. This comes down to the mistake of treating wilderness areas, as Simon and Alagona put it, as "islands of nature surrounded by a sea of development." It's all fine and dandy that we try not to leave a trace as we explore our national parks and any other natural environments. But we can't forget about the environmental impacts we cause elsewhere. Making conscientious purchasing choices, buying only the equipment and clothing you need and caring for it so that it lasts as long as possible, means that there's less impact where these goods are produced.

Increased consumption means increased production. And what goes with it: increased environmental impacts. Through our buying choices, we might leave no trace in our favorite wilderness areas, but we do leave a trace elsewhere. Is our relationship with nature respectful if we treat one place as a treasure and another as a dumpster?

This effect isn't limited to outdoor equipment alone. All that we buy and consume comes with an environmental cost when it's produced, distributed, and later disposed of. This is what *Beyond Leave No Trace* is about. Instead of thinking merely about the direct impacts of our activity in the natural environment, we also need to think about our global footprint. In our modern, urbanized world, it's impossible to stop consumption. It's unrealistic to assume that we'll stop striving to interact with nature through a variety of activities that require equipment. And it would be a classic example of the pot calling the kettle black to deem as hypocrites nature lovers who contribute to the problem by purchasing outdoor equipment. We all have a footprint, if not through buying a high-tech jacket or a surfboard, then through other purchases, including our daily groceries.

Joan Maloof, the director of forest conservation non-profit Old-Growth Forest Network, writes in her book *Teaching the Trees: Lessons from the Forest* that "it is a paradox we must live with: even when we try to do the right thing we sometimes destroy habitat. But all animals do that when making their homes—living on the earth requires harming other organisms. I have come to believe that the only moral solution to the paradox is to strive to minimize our impacts and to be utterly clear about the impacts we are having."

As a nature lover who cares about the environment, I faced the same dilemma when I started surfing. Surfers might appear to be an environmentally conscious crowd, but traditional wetsuits and surfboards are made of toxic materials. They cause impact when they're manufactured, used, and disposed of. A big challenge in the industry is how to recycle them.

I fell in love with surfing, but I didn't love the fact that my activity would be so harmful to the environment. To reduce my impact, I chose to buy a wetsuit made of an emerging, more environmentally friendly material called Yulex (currently only offered by Patagonia) that's 85 percent natural rubber from sustainable sources. My purchasing choice still made an environmental impact (let's not hide this fact), but a lower one than buying a traditional neoprene wetsuit. I also managed to lower my impact when buying a surfboard. Modern surfboards are made of harmful, synthetic materials. Fortunately, companies are turning to eco-friendly solutions. One of them is a French company, Notox, which manufactures boards made of cork. I bought one and am happy not only because it has a smaller footprint, but also because it's a great product made by a small, eco-conscious company that shares my values.

I don't fool myself into thinking that my purchasing choices were 100 percent green. Everything we consume has an impact. As Joan Maloof suggests, the best we can do is strive to reduce our impact and be aware that we do have an impact no matter what we do. At the same time, our purchases can bring us closer to nature and through this deeper bond, inspire us to protect it. Surfing has made me appreciate the beauty and significance of the ocean, which was previously difficult for me, a person born and living in a non-coastal city, to understand.

One of my favorite outdoor equipment companies, Patagonia, writes in its mission statement: "Our criteria for the best product rests on function, repairability, and, foremost, durability. Among the most direct ways we can limit ecological impacts is with goods that last for generations or can be recycled so the materials in them remain in use. Making the best product matters for saving the planet."[170]

For us consumers, making sure that we really need something, and if we deem we do, buying the best product so that we can use it for as long as possible, represents a moral obligation. We need to make sure that not only we, but also future generations can get to enjoy interactions with nature both wild and urban.

If you want to learn more about nature stewardship, visit my website at *www.MartinSummerAuthor.com*, head to book resources and access additional content by typing the password "connecting."

Let's Not Forget About Each Other

I once went on a quick bike ride to a local forest. It was a chilly, windy winter morning with few people outside. The deeper into the forest I went, the less likely it was I would meet someone. It wasn't a nice day to be out, and it wasn't a popular spot. But surprisingly, on a rarely frequented mossy trail among pine trees, I met a man walking his dog. The simple "hello" we exchanged wasn't a mere meaningless courtesy. His wide smile said more than that. Despite passing the stranger in a few seconds, I felt a deep connection with him. We were the only two humans (plus a dog) around. Each of us enjoyed the forest despite the less-than-ideal weather. There was a quiet understanding between us, a fleeting expression of mutual respect and shared interests.

Nature can help us get close to each other as we realize that others love the natural environment as much as we do. It can also remind us that we're all a part of something bigger than us. This is another key aspect of stewardship we shouldn't forget. Humans are also a part of nature. As such, we owe respect to fellow human beings we encounter on our outings. It doesn't change whether we're at a small local park, an urban beach, a national park, or any other wild area. It doesn't matter whether they're fellow hikers, surfers, climbers, skiers, or people sitting on a bench enjoying the nature around. This is the role we take on as nature stewards: to protect and respect the world around us, including all of its inhabitants. By working together and through mutual respect we can do wonders for the environment—so let's do that!

Conclusion

ᵃ⁂

Exploring the wild and remote landscapes of Kyrgyzstan wasn't an easy trip for my girlfriend and me. The language barrier posed a constant challenge. It started right at the airport where a salesclerk selling tourist SIM cards didn't speak English. Our rental car needed a mechanic on our second day (fortunately, we were still close to Bishkek, the nation's capital, and help could come quickly). Wild camping (it was the first time we tried it) was at first a terrifying experience. In the beginning, no phone reception for most of the trip outside of the major towns and cities was also stressful.

As we drove the country's potholed roads, bought food at local markets (if you're ever in Kyrgyzstan or neighboring countries, definitely stuff yourself with lepyoshka, local leavened bread), and experienced semi-nomadic lifestyles so different to what we were used to in Europe, we eventually fell into a simple rhythm. We woke up in a tent or in a car parked somewhere in a remote area, took care of daily hygiene, and set off to explore further. We used the conveniences of modern living—an off-road vehicle, some travel equipment, and technology (the local SIM card proved useful to plan ahead and communicate with loved ones) to connect with wild, remote nature on a deeper level. Thanks to progress, exploring the world is much easier today than it was hundreds of years ago. But, at the same time, there's less wilderness to explore, which brings us to the conclusion of this book.

The trends are clear. Each year, more people move to cities. More and more areas around the world become urban, replacing previously rural areas. The urban sprawl is yet another sad sign of modern times. Access to wild, pristine nature is getting more difficult, particularly for those who live and work in big cities. However, this doesn't mean that we nature lovers should give up our love and accept that the world is turning into one big chunk of concrete and asphalt.

Quite the contrary: nature-loving urbanites should strive to be even more connected to it. We need to set the right example for those who are detached from it and have spent their entire lives in our urban jungles. Through expressing our love for the natural environment and encouraging others to experience it with us—even if it's a brief, but focused walk in a local urban park—we can become a force for good. We can teach city dwellers the importance and joy of exploring natural and semi-natural habitats. If not us, who *is* going to inspire and educate about the value of the wild?

We've explored the many risks associated with urban living. We can mitigate many of them through increased awareness of how they affect our everyday lives. We can also implement some simple fixes and habits. When we combine these strategies with daily natural exposure—you've learned that small doses do exist even in the biggest cities—we'll achieve what you might have considered impossible before reading this book. We gain the ability to stay close to nature in our rapidly urbanizing world.

This, however, doesn't mean we can do away with the wilderness. I strove to provide advice that's available to anyone regardless of their financial status or time available. At the same time, I encourage you include in your budget and schedule regular extended stays in nature of at least several focused hours. It might sound like an unnecessary luxury. After all, who has time and/or money to afford a trip or disconnect for a few long hours? But as the old saying goes, where there's a will there's a way. Natural environment is our natural human habitat. We might no longer want to live without the modern conveniences (understandably so), but periodically returning to our roots can provide life-changing experiences worth so much more than they cost.

In wild nature we can forget about the fast pace of our modern lives, the demands on our time, and the responsibilities we bear on our shoulders. We can gain perspective on how insignificant we are in the grand scheme of things.

While that may sound depressing, remember it's actually a good thing. We gain humility and appreciation of life when we realize our smallness. We can heal our psychological traumas as we get away from it all and make our lives simple again. We can benefit from this effect while going on a multi-day hike. We can recover by spending a night in a spartan cabin in the woods. Exploring the open seas on a sailboat can change us, too. So can enjoying the ocean on a stand-up paddle board, or sitting in an inspiring surrounding taking in the views.

Nature is a precious gift we might not fully appreciate as we spend most of our days in air-conditioned buildings. So, let's make a conscious effort to expose ourselves to it in doses both small and large.

Thank you for taking your time to read my book. I hope I've inspired you to try to see nature all around you. I wish you an abundance of beautiful, memorable moments wherever you find yourself. Please visit my website *www.MartinSummerAuthor.com* for more information about my work, additional resources, and updates about my new projects. I will also greatly appreciate you telling other people about my book or reviewing it on your favorite online bookstore.

About the Author

Martin writes about the natural environment and the relationship we have with it. His books aim to encourage his readers to embrace the philosophy of biophilia, the innate need humans have to connect with other life forms. Passionate about outdoor sports, traveling, and learning, he seeks practical answers to the question of how we can live better through getting closer to nature.

References

1   Allan, J. R., Venter, O., & Watson, J. E. (2017). Temporally inter-comparable maps of terrestrial wilderness and the Last of the Wild. *Scientific Data*, 4(1). doi: 10.1038/sdata.2017.187

2   Crowther, T., Glick, H., Covey, K. et al. (2015). Mapping tree density at a global scale. *Nature*, 525, 201–205. doi: 10.1038/nature14967

3   van den Bosch, M., Sang, A. O. (2017). Urban natural environments as nature-based solutions for improved public health. A systematic review of reviews. *Environmental Research*, 58, 373–384. doi: 10.1016/j.envres.2017.05.040

4   Maas, J., Verheij, R. A., Groenewegen, P. P., de Vries, S., Spreeuwenberg, P. (2006). Green space, urbanity, and health: How strong is the relation? *Journal of Epidemiology & Community Health*, 60(7), 587–592.

5   Bratman, G. N., Daily, G. C., Levy, B. J., and Gross, J. J. (2015). The benefits of nature experience: improved affect and cognition. *Landscape and Urban Planning*, 138, 41–50. doi: 10.1016/j.landurbplan.2015.02.005

6   Barton, J., Pretty, J. (2010). What is the best dose of nature and green exercise for improving mental health? A multi-study analysis. *Environmental Science and Technology*, 44, 3947–3955. doi: 10.1021/es903183r

7   Hartig, T., Kaiser, F., Strumse, E. (2007). Psychological restoration in nature as a source of motivation for ecological behaviour. *Environmental Conservation*, 34(4), 291—299. doi: 10.1017/S0376892907004250

8   Yan, W. (2016, April 4). *The Prehistoric Secrets of Olduvai Gorge.* JSTOR Daily. Retrieved from https://daily.jstor.org/prehistoric-secrets-of-olduvai-gorge/

9   Cerling, T. E., Mbua, E., Kirera, F. M., Manthi, F. K., Grine, F. E., Leakey, M. G., Sponheimer, M., Uno, K. T. (2011). Diet of Paranthropus boisei in the early Pleistocene of East Africa. *Proceedings of the National Academy of Sciences of the United States of America*, 108(23), 9337–9341. doi: 10.1073/pnas.1104627108

10   University of Colorado Denver (2013, December 5.) *Discovery of partial skeleton suggests ruggedly built, tree-climbing human ancestor.* Retrieved from https://phys .org/news/2013-12-discovery-partial-skeleton-ruggedly-built.html

11   Bates, Todd. B. (2016, March 9). *Early Human Habitat, Recreated for First Time, Shows Life Was No Picnic.* Retrieved from https://news.rutgers.edu/feature/ early-human-*habitat*-recreated-first-time-shows-life-was-no-picnic/20160309#. XhQW4Px7lPY

12   Gowlett, J. (2016). The discovery of fire by humans: A long and convoluted process. *Philosophical Transactions of The Royal Society of London. Series B. Biological Sciences,* 371(1696). doi: 10.1098/rstb.2015.0164

13   Stokes Brown, C. (n.d.). *Foraging.* Retrieved from https://www.khanacademy. org/partner-content/big-history-project/early-humans/how-did-first-humans -live/a/foraging

14   Lee, R. B., Heywood, D. R. (1999). *The Cambridge Encyclopedia of Hunters and Gatherers.* Cambridge University Press.

15   Scherjon, F., Bakels, C., MacDonald, K., Roebroeks, W. (2015). Burning the Land: An Ethnographic Study of Off-Site Fire Use by Current and Historically Documented Foragers and Implications for the Interpretation of Past Fire Practices in the Landscape. *Current Anthropology,* 56(3), 299—326. doi: 10.1086/681561

16   Smith, F. A., Smith, R. E., Lyons, S. K., Payne, J. L. (2018). Body size downgrading of mammals over the late Quaternary. *Science,* 360(6386), 310–313. doi:10.1126/science.aao5987

17   United Nations (2018). *The speed of urbanization around the world.* Retrieved from https://population.un.org/wup/Publications/

18   Angel, J. L. (1969). The bases of paleodemography. *American Journal of Physical Anthropology,* 30(3), 427–437. doi:10.1002/ajpa.1330300314

19   The World Bank (2019). Life expectancy at birth, total (years). Retrieved from https://data.worldbank.org/indicator/SP.DYN.LE00.IN

20   Buchwald, E. (2018, September 21). *Outdoor recreation is a more than $400 billion industry.* Retrieved from https://www.marketwatch.com/story/outdoor -recreation-is-a-more-than-400-billion-industry-2018-09-21

21   Terrapin Bright Green (2014, May 1). *The Economics of Biophilia.* Retrieved from https://www.terrapinbrightgreen.com/reports/the-economics-of-biophilia/

22 Ritchie, H., Roser, M. (2019). *Urbanization*. Retrieved from: https://ourworldindata.org/urbanization

23 Callaway, E. (2017). Oldest Homo sapiens fossil claim rewrites our species history. *Nature*. doi: 10.1038/nature.2017.22114

24 Torrey, B. B. (2004, April 23). *Urbanization: An Environmental Force to Be Reckoned With*. Retrieved from https://www.prb.org/urbanization-an -environmental-force-to-be-reckoned-with/

25 McDonald, R. I. et al. (2020). Research gaps in knowledge of the impact of urban growth on biodiversity. *Nature Sustainability*, 3(16–24). doi: 10.1038/ s41893-019-0436-6

26 PersilUK (2016). *Free the Kids - Dirt is Good*. Retrieved from https://www.youtube.com/watch?v=8Q2WnCkBTw0

27 Sarigiannis, D. A. (Ed.) World Health Organization (2013). *Combined or multiple exposure to health stressors in indoor built environments*. Retrieved from http://www.euro.who.int/en/health-topics/environment-and-health/air-quality /publications/2014/combined-or-multiple-exposure-to-health-stressors-in -indoor-built-environments

28 U.S. Environmental Protection Agency. 1989. *Report to Congress on indoor air quality: Volume 2*. EPA/400/1-89/001C. Washington, DC.

29 U.S. Environmental Protection Agency. *Report on the Environment. Indoor Air Quality*. Retrieved from https://www.epa.gov/report-environment/indoor-air -quality.

30 U.S. Environmental Protection Agency. *Indoor Air Quality (IAQ). Indoor Pollutants and Sources*. Retrieved from https://www.epa.gov/indoor-air-quality -iaq/indoor-pollutants-and-sources

31 Kilpeläinen, M., Terho, E. O., Helenius, H., Koskenvuo, M. (2001). Home dampness, current allergic diseases, and respiratory infections among young adults. *Thorax*, 56(6), 462—467. doi: 10.1136/thorax.56.6.462

32 Pica, N., Bouvier, N. M. (2012). Environmental Factors Affecting the Transmission of Respiratory Viruses. *Current Opinion in Virology*, 2(1): 90–95. doi: 10.1016/j.coviro.2011.12.003

33 Robson, D. (2015, October 19). *The real reason germs spread in the winter*. Retrieved from https://www.bbc.com/future/article/20151016-the-real-reason -germs-spread-in-the-winter

34   Kuo, M. (2015). How might contact with nature promote human health? Promising mechanisms and a possible central pathway. *Frontiers in Psychology*, 6, 1093. doi: 10.3389/fpsyg.2015.01093

35   Roenneberg, T., Wirz-Justice, A., Merrow, M. (2003). Life between Clocks: Daily Temporal Patterns of Human Chronotypes. *Journal of Biological Rhythms*, 18(1), 80–90. doi: 10.1177/0748730402239679.

36   Challet, E. (2013). Circadian Clocks, Food Intake, and Metabolism. *Progress in Molecular Biology and Translational Science*, 119, 105—135. doi: 10.1016/B978-0-12-396971-2.00005-1

37   van Someren, E. J., Riemersma-Van Der Lek, R. F. (2007). Live to the rhythm, slave to the rhythm. *Sleep Medicine Reviews*, 11(6), 465–484. doi: 10.1016/j.smrv.2007.07.003

38   Harb, F., Hidalgo, M. P., Martau, B. (2015) Lack of exposure to natural light in the workspace is associated with physiological, sleep and depressive symptoms. *Chronobiology International*, 32(3), 368–375. doi: 10.3109/07420528.2014.982757

39   Kuehn, B. M. (2017). Resetting the Circadian Clock Might Boost Metabolic Health. *JAMA*, 317(13), 1303–1305. doi:10.1001/jama.2017.0653

40   Matheson, A., O'Brien, L., Reid, J.-A. (2014), The impact of shiftwork on health: a literature review. *Journal of Clinical Nursing*, 23, 3309–3320. doi: 10.1111/jocn.12524

41   Folkard, S. (2008). Do Permanent Night Workers Show Circadian Adjustment? A Review Based on the Endogenous Melatonin Rhythm. *Chronobiology International*, 25(2), 215–224. doi: 10.1080/07420520802106835

42   The National Optical Astronomy Observatory (NOAO). *Recommended Light Levels*. Retrieved from https://www.noao.edu/education/QLTkit/ACTIVITY _Documents/Safety/LightLevels_outdoor+indoor.pdf

43   Bureau of Labor Statistics, U.S. Department of Labor, The Economics Daily. *Over 90 percent of protective service and construction and extraction jobs require work outdoors*. Retrieved from https://www.bls.gov/opub/ted/2017/over-90 -percent-of-protective-service-and-construction-and-extraction-jobs-require -work-outdoors.htm

44   Holick, M. F. (2011). *The Vitamin D Solution: A 3-Step Strategy to Cure Our Most Common Health Problems*. Plume.

45   Bell, T. D., Demay, M. B., Burnett-Bowie, S.-A. M. (2010). The biology and
      pathology of vitamin D control in bone. *Journal of Cellular Biochemistry*, 111(1),
      7–13. doi: 10.1002/jcb.22661

46   Watkins, R. R., Lemonovich, T. L., Salata, R. A. (2015). An update on the
      association of vitamin D deficiency with common infectious diseases. *Canadian
      Journal of Physiology and Pharmacology*, 93(5), 363–368. doi: 10.1139/cjpp-
      2014-0352

47   Angeline, M. E., Gee, A. O., Shindle, M., Warren, R. F., & Rodeo, S. A.
      (2013). The Effects of Vitamin D Deficiency in Athletes. *The American Journal
      of Sports Medicine*, 41(2), 461–464. doi: 10.1177/0363546513475787

48   Roecklein, K. A., Rohan, K. J. (2005). Seasonal Affective Disorder. *Psychiatry
      (Edgmont)*, 2(1), 20–26. PMID: 21179639

49   Avery, D. H., Kizer, D., Bolte, M. A., Hellekson, C. (2001). Bright light
      therapy of subsyndromal seasonal affective disorder in the workplace: morning
      vs. afternoon exposure. *Acta Psychiatrica Scandinavica*, 103, 267–274. doi:
      10.1034/j.1600-0447.2001.00078.x

50   Workman, L. (2014, October 27). *SAD: debilitating condition or evolutionary
      survival strategy?* Retrieved from https://weather.com/en-GB/unitedkingdom
      /health/news/sad-debilitating-condition-or-evolutionary-survival
      -strategy-20141027

51   Nussbaumer-Streit, B., Winkler, D., Spies, M., Kasper, S., Pjrek, E. (2017).
      Prevention of seasonal affective disorder in daily clinical practice: results of a
      survey in German-speaking countries. *BMC Psychiatry*, 17(1). doi: 10.1186/
      s12888-017-1403-2

52   Dolgin, E. (2015, March 18). The Myopia Boom. *Nature*, 519(7543), 276–278.
      doi: 10.1038/519276a.

53   Blackwell, D. L., Clarke, T. C. (2018). State Variation in Meeting the 2008
      Federal Guidelines for Both Aerobic and Muscle-strengthening Activities
      Through Leisure-time Physical Activity Among Adults Aged 18–64: United
      States, 2010–2015. *National Health Statistics Reports*, 112, 1—22.

54   Eurostat. *How much do Europeans exercise?* Retrieved from https://ec.europa.eu
      /eurostat/web/products-eurostat-news/-/DDN-20170302-1

55   Harvey, H. (2017, July 30). *Dreaming of moving to the country? Don't say I didn't
      warn you.* Retrieved from https://www.telegraph.co.uk/women/life/dreaming
      -moving-country-dont-say-didnt-warn/

56   Parks, S. E. (2003). Differential correlates of physical activity in urban and rural adults of various socioeconomic backgrounds in the United States. *Journal of Epidemiology & Community Health*, 57(1), 29–35. doi: 10.1136/jech.57.1.29

57   *The Indoor Generation* (2018). Retrieved from https://www.velux.com /indoorgeneration

58   Cummings, B. E., Waring, M. S. (2019). Potted plants do not improve indoor air quality: a review and analysis of reported VOC removal efficiencies. *Journal of Exposure Science & Environmental Epidemiology*. doi: 10.1038/s41370-019-0175-9

59   Avery, D. H., Kizer, D., Bolte, M. A., Hellekson, C. (2001). Bright light therapy of subsyndromal seasonal affective disorder in the workplace: morning vs. afternoon exposure. *Acta Psychiatrica Scandinavica*, 103, 267–274. doi: 10.1034/j.1600-0447.2001.00078.x

60   Ulmer, A. (2020, March 23). *Indians breathe easier as lockdowns to halt coronavirus clear smog*. Retrieved from https://www.reuters.com/article/us -health-coronavirus-india-pollution/indians-breathe-easier-as-lockdowns-to -halt-coronavirus-clear-smog-idUSKBN21A1BV

61   World Health Organization (2014, March 25). *7 million premature deaths annually linked to air pollution*. Retrieved from https://www.who.int /mediacentre/news/releases/2014/air-pollution/en/

62   Burnett, R.T. et al. (2018). Global estimates of mortality associated with long-term exposure to outdoor fine particulate matter. *Proceedings of the National Academy of Sciences of the United States of America*, 115(38), 9592–9597. doi: 10.1073/pnas.1803222115

63   Vidal, J. (2016, May 12). *Air pollution rising at an 'alarming rate' in world's cities*. Retrieved from https://www.theguardian.com/environment/2016/may/12/air -pollution-rising-at-an-alarming-rate-in-worlds-cities

64   Ibid.

65   India Today (2019, November 1). *How does air pollution affect health? These 9 studies show the horrifying reality*. Retrieved from https://www.indiatoday.in /education-today/gk-current-affairs/story/how-does-air-pollution-affect-health -these-9-studies-show-the-horrifying-reality-1614883-2019-11-01

66   FP Staff (2019, November 5). *Delhi Air Pollution Updates*. Retrieved from https://www.firstpost.com/india/delhi-air-pollution-highlights-updates-odd -even-scheme-2019-today-smog-air-quality-index-haryana-punjab-ncr-aqi -latest-news-health-minister-7592981.html

67 World Health Organization (2014, March 25). *7 million premature deaths annually linked to air pollution.* Retrieved from https://www.who.int /mediacentre/news/releases/2014/air-pollution/en/

68 Strosnider, H., Kennedy, C., Monti, M., Yip, F. (2017). Rural and Urban Differences in Air Quality, 2008–2012, and Community Drinking Water Quality, 2010–2015 — United States. *Surveillance Summaries*, 66(13), 1–10. doi:10.15585/mmwr.ss6613a1

69 BBC News (2017, January 6). *Is it healthier to live in the countryside?* Retrieved from https://www.bbc.com/news/health-38520092

70 Cichowicz, R., Stelęgowski, A. (2019). Average Hourly Concentrations of Air Contaminants in Selected Urban, Town, and Rural Sites. *Archives of Environmental Contamination and Toxicology*, 77(2), 197–213. doi: 10.1007/ s00244-019-00627-8

71 Michigan State University (2016, January 21). *The air we breathe: Studying the impact of air pollution in rural environments.* Retrieved from https://www.canr .msu.edu/news/the_air_we_breathe_studying_the_impact_of_air_pollution_in _rural_environmen

72 Smith, C. (2018, May 31). *How to use your garden to fight pollution.* Retrieved from https://www.gold.ac.uk/news/phyto-sensor/

73 Schlesinger, W. H. (2017, April 6). *Trees and Air Pollution.* Retrieved from https://blog.nature.org/science/2017/04/06/trees-air-pollution-balance -ecosystem-services-ozone/

74 Laskowski, E. R. (2017, April 12). *Does air pollution make outdoor exercise risky? What if you have asthma or another health problem?* Retrieved from https://www .mayoclinic.org/healthy-lifestyle/fitness/expert-answers/air-pollution-and -exercise/faq-20058563

75 Carrington, D. (2017, June 14). *Side street routes to avoid city pollution can cut exposure by half.* Retrieved from https://www.theguardian.com /environment/2017/jun/14/side-street-routes-avoid-city-pollution-cut-exposure -by-half

76 Health Effects Institute (2010). *Traffic-Related Air Pollution: A Critical Review of the Literature on Emissions, Exposure, and Health Effects.* Retrieved from https: //www.healtheffects.org/publication/traffic-related-air-pollution-critical-review -literature-emissions-exposure-and-health

77 Cecil, N. (2014, May 8). *Walk away from kerb to avoid fumes in London, adviser urges*. Retrieved from https://www.standard.co.uk/news/london/walk-away-from -kerb-to-avoid-fumes-in-london-adviser-urges-9335615.html

78 Lim, C. C. et al. (2019). Mediterranean Diet and the Association Between Air Pollution and Cardiovascular Disease Mortality Risk. *Circulation*, 139(15), 1766–1775. doi: 10.1161/CIRCULATIONAHA.118.035742

79 Sifferlin, A. (2018, May 21). *Can Your Diet Reduce the Effects of Air Pollution? Here's What a New Study Says*. Retrieved from https://time.com/5285664 /mediterranean-diet-air-pollution/

80 Klein, K. (2016, December 23). *In a Noisy World, Our Brains Still Need the Sounds of Nature*. Retrieved from https://www.alleghenyfront.org/in-a-noisy -world-our-brains-still-need-the-sounds-of-nature/

81 HealthLink BC. *Harmful Noise Levels*. Retrieved from https://www.healthlinkbc .ca/health-topics/tf4173

82 Center for Hearing and Communication. *Common environmental noise levels*. Retrieved from https://chchearing.org/noise/common-environmental-noise -levels/

83 Ibid.

84 Zielinski, S. (2011, November 3). *Secrets of a Lion's Roar*. Retrieved from https: //www.smithsonianmag.com/science-nature/secrets-of-a-lions-roar-126395997/

85 Podos, J., Cohn-Haft, M. (2019). Extremely loud mating songs at close range in white bellbirds. *Current Biology*, 29(20). doi: 10.1016/j.cub.2019.09.028

86 Mimi Hearing Technologies (2017, March 8). *Worldwide Hearing Index 2017*. Retrieved from https://www.mimi.io/en/blog/2017/3/8/worldwide-hearing -index-2017

87 Paul, K. C., Haan, M., Mayeda, E. R., Ritz, B. R. (2019). Ambient Air Pollution, Noise, and Late-Life Cognitive Decline and Dementia Risk. *Annual Review of Public Health*, 40(1), 203–220. doi: 10.1146/annurev-publhealth-040218-044058

88 Münzel, T., Schmidt, F. P., Steven, S., Herzog, J., Daiber, A., Sørensen, M. (2018). Environmental Noise and the Cardiovascular System. *Journal of the American College of Cardiology*. 71(6), 688–697. doi: 10.1016/j. jacc.2017.12.015

89   Alberti, P. W. (1992). Noise induced hearing loss. *BMJ*, 304(6826), 522. doi: 10.1136/bmj.304.6826.522

90   Hammer, M. S., Swinburn, T. K., Neitzel, R. L. (2014). Environmental Noise Pollution in the United States: Developing an Effective Public Health Response. *Environmental Health Perspectives*, 122(2). doi: 10.1289/ehp.1307272

91   European Environment Agency (2019). *Exposure of Europe's population to environmental noise*. Retrieved from https://www.eea.europa.eu/data-and-maps /indicators/exposure-to-and-annoyance-by-2/assessment-4

92   The National Institute for Occupational Safety and Health (NIOSH). *Noise and Hearing Loss Prevention*. Retrieved from https://www.cdc.gov/niosh/topics/noise /default.html

93   Center for Hearing and Communication. *Common environmental noise levels*. Retrieved from https://chchearing.org/noise/common-environmental-noise -levels/

94   Patel, S. S. (2018, August 10). *Are You Listening? Hear What Uninterrupted Silence Sounds Like*. Retrieved from https://www.npr .org/2018/08/10/633201540/are-you-listening-hear-what-uninterrupted -silence-sounds-like

95   Barone, J. (2009, July 24). *What Do Urban Sounds Do to Your Brain?* Retrieved from https://www.discovermagazine.com/mind/what-do-urban-sounds-do-to -your-brain

96   Kunc, H. P., Schmidt, R. (2019). The effects of anthropogenic noise on animals: a meta-analysis. *Biology Letters*, 15(11), 20190649. doi: 10.1098/rsbl.2019.0649

97   Alvarsson, J. J., Wiens, S., Nilsson, M. E. (2010). Stress Recovery during Exposure to Nature Sound and Environmental Noise. *International Journal of Environmental Research and Public Health*, 7(3), 1036–1046. doi: 10.3390/ ijerph7031036

98   Beutel, M. E. et al. (2016). Noise Annoyance Is Associated with Depression and Anxiety in the General Population—The Contribution of Aircraft Noise. *Plos One*, 11(5). doi: 10.1371/journal.pone.0155357

99   National Park Service (2017, December 5). *Mapping Sound*. Retrieved from https://www.nps.gov/subjects/sound/soundmap.htm

100   European Environment Agency. *The NOISE Observation & Information Service for Europe*. Retrieved from http://noise.eea.europa.eu/

101 Sharkey, J. (2008, August 30). *Helping the Stars Take Back the Night.* Retrieved from https://www.nytimes.com/2008/08/31/business/31essay.html

102 Cho, Y., Ryu, S.-H., Lee, B. R., Kim, K. H., Lee, E., & Choi, J. (2015). Effects of artificial light at night on human health: A literature review of observational and experimental studies applied to exposure assessment. *Chronobiology International*, 32(9), 1294–1310. doi: 10.3109/07420528.2015.1073158

103 Falchi, F., Cinzano, P., Duriscoe, D., Kyba, C. C. M., Elvidge, C. D., Baugh, K., … Furgoni, R. (2016). The new world atlas of artificial night sky brightness. *Science Advances*, 2(6). doi: 10.1126/sciadv.1600377

104 Ibid.

105 Dunham, W. (2017, November 22). *The future looks bright: light pollution rises on a global scale.* Retrieved from https://www.reuters.com/article/us-science-light -idUSKBN1DM2OK

106 Drake, N. (2019, April 3). *Our nights are getting brighter, and Earth is paying the price.* Retrieved from https://www.nationalgeographic.com/science/2019/04 /nights-are-getting-brighter-earth-paying-the-price-light-pollution-dark-skies/

107 International Dark-Sky Association. *International Dark Sky Communities.* Retrieved from https://www.darksky.org/our-work/conservation/idsp /communities/

108 International Dark-Sky Association. *International Dark Sky Parks.* Retrieved from https://www.darksky.org/our-work/conservation/idsp/parks/

109 Chang, A.-M., Aeschbach, D., Duffy, J. F., Czeisler, C. A. (2014). Evening use of light-emitting eReaders negatively affects sleep, circadian timing, and next-morning alertness. *Proceedings of the National Academy of Sciences of the United States of America*, 112(4), 1232–1237. doi: 10.1073/pnas.1418490112

110 International Dark-Sky Association. *Outdoor Lighting Basics.* Retrieved from https://www.darksky.org/our-work/lighting/lighting-for-citizens/lighting-basics/

111 Ro, C. (2019, October 9). Dunbar's number: *Why we can only maintain 150 relationships.* Retrieved from https://www.bbc.com/future/article/20191001 -dunbars-number-why-we-can-only-maintain-150-relationships

112 Smith, L. (2018, June 19). *All the Ways Living in a City Messes With Your Mental Health.* Retrieved from https://www.vice.com/en_us/article/qvnngm/all-the -ways-living-in-a-city-messes-with-your-mental-health

113 Kennedy, D. P., Gläscher, J., Tyszka, J. M., Adolphs, R. (2009). Personal space regulation by the human amygdala. *Nature Neuroscience*, 12(10), 1226–1227. doi: 10.1038/nn.2381

114 Sorokowska, A. et al. (2017). Preferred Interpersonal Distances: A Global Comparison. Journal of Cross-Cultural Psychology, 48(4), 577–592. doi: 10.1177/0022022117698039

115 Bowman, K. (2016). *Movement Matters: Essays on Movement Science, Movement Ecology, and the Nature of Movement.* Propriometrics Press.

116 Krisciunas, K., Carona, D. (2015). At What Distance Can the Human Eye Detect a Candle Flame? Cornell University Library, arXiv:1507.06270

117 National Park Service (2020, January 15). *Wilderness Permits.* Retrieved from https://www.nps.gov/yose/planyourvisit/wildpermits.htm

118 National Park Service (2019, May 6). *Backcountry Advance Reservations.* Retrieved from https://www.nps.gov/glac/planyourvisit/backcountry -reservations.htm

119 Walmsley, D. J., Lewis, G. J. (1989). The Pace of Pedestrian Flows in Cities. *Environment and Behavior*, 21(2), 123–150. doi: 10.1177/0013916589212001

120 Wiseman, R. *Welcome to the Pace of Life Project.* Retrieved from http://www .richardwiseman.com/quirkology/pace_home.htm

121 Levine, R. V., Norenzayan, A. (1999). The Pace of Life in 31 Countries. *Journal of Cross-Cultural Psychology*, 30(2), 178–205. doi: 10.1177/0022022199030002003

122 Caldwell, L. L. (2005). Leisure and health: why is leisure therapeutic? *British Journal of Guidance & Counselling*, 33(1), 7–26. doi: 10.1080/03069880412331335939

123 Hribernik, J., Mussap, A. J. (2010). Research note: Leisure satisfaction and subjective wellbeing. *Annals of Leisure Research*, 13(4), 701–708. doi: 10.1080/11745398.2010.9686871

124 Brajša-Žganec, A., Merkaš, M., Šverko, I. (2010). Quality of Life and Leisure Activities: How do Leisure Activities Contribute to Subjective Well-Being? *Social Indicators Research*, 102(1), 81–91. doi: 10.1007/s11205-010-9724-2

125 Brown, S. (n.d.) *What makes SPEED an addiction?* Retrieved from http://www .stephaniebrownphd.com/what-makes-speed-an-addiction/

126 Murphy, K. (2014, July 25). *No Time to Think.* Retrieved from https://www
.nytimes.com/2014/07/27/sunday-review/no-time-to-think.html

127 World Cities Culture Forum. % *of public green space (parks and gardens).*
Retrieved from http://www.worldcitiescultureforum.com/data/of-public-green
-space-parks-and-gardens

128 Ibid.

129 Treepedia. Retrieved from http://senseable.mit.edu/treepedia

130 Teirstein, Z. (2018, May 31*). Hawaii's rarest plants are in crisis. Meet the people
fighting to save them.* Retrieved from https://grist.org/article/hawaiis-rarest
-plants-are-in-crisis-meet-the-people-fighting-to-save-them/

131 Cronon, W. (1996). The Trouble with Wilderness: Or, Getting Back to the
Wrong Nature. *Environmental History,* 1(1), 7. doi: 10.2307/3985059

132 Brown, S. (2014, August 4). *Reflections on Kate Murphy's article, "No Time to
Think" in the NYTimes, Sunday Review,* July 27, 2014. Retrieved from http:
//www.stephaniebrownphd.com/reflections-article/

133 BBC News (2012, September 10). *Who What Why: Why are there so many
seagulls in cities?* Retrieved from https://www.bbc.com/news
/magazine-19490866

134 Curtis, R. (1999). *Outdoor Action Guide to Nature Observation & Stalking.*
Retrieved from https://www.princeton.edu/~oa/nature/naturobs.shtml

135 Stork, N. E., Mcbroom, J., Gely, C., Hamilton, A. J. (2015). New approaches
narrow global species estimates for beetles, insects, and terrestrial arthropods.
Proceedings of the National Academy of Sciences, 112(24), 7519–7523. doi:
10.1073/pnas.1502408112

136 Mcgann, J. P. (2017). Poor human olfaction is a 19th-century myth. *Science,*
356(6338). doi: 10.1126/science.aam7263

137 McCartney, S. (2017, May 15). *The nose has it: it's no surprise humans' sense of
smell can be as good as dogs'.* Retrieved from https://www.theguardian.com
/commentisfree/2017/may/15/nose-human-sense-smell-rival-dogs-perfumer

138 Palermo, E. (2013, June 21). *Why Does Rain Smell Good?* Retrieved from
https://www.livescience.com/37648-good-smells-rain-petrichor.html

139 Villazon, L. (n.d.). *Why does the sea smell like the sea?* Retrieved from https:
//www.sciencefocus.com/planet-earth/why-does-the-sea-smell-like-the-sea/

140 Discovery News (2014, January 14). *Why Cold Air Smells Different.* Retrieved from https://www.seeker.com/why-cold-air-smells-different-1768222636.html

141 Rosenbaum, S. (2013, July 17). *Ooooh, that smell! Odors rise with the temperature.* Retrieved from https://www.nbcnews.com/news/us-news/ooooh -smell-odors-rise-temperature-flna6C10663511

142 Pinsker, J. (2017, October 5). *What Do Professional Apple Farmers Think of People Who Pick Apples for Fun?* Retrieved from https://www.theatlantic.com /business/archive/2015/11/what-do-professional-apple-farmers-think-of-people -who-pick-apples-for-fun/414382/

143 Guertner, M. (n.d.). *Losæter: Urban farming in Oslo.* Retrieved from https: //www.visitoslo.com/en/your-oslo/oslo-for-foodies/urban-farming/

144 http://fifthquarternorwich.weebly.com/

145 Zipfel, B., Berger, L. (2007). Shod versus unshod: The emergence of forefoot pathology in modern humans? *The Foot*, 17(4), 205–213. doi: 10.1016/j. foot.2007.06.002

146 Sternbergh, A. (2008, April 18). *How We're Wrecking Our Feet With Every Step We Take.* Retrieved from https://nymag.com/health/features/46213/

147 Florio, G. (2018, June 25). *Meet Animal Flow, the Workout That's About to Take Over the Fitness World* Retrieved from https://www.popsugar.com/fitness/What -Animal-Flow-44369195

148 Huttunen, P., Kokko, L., Ylijukuri, V. (2004). Winter swimming improves general well-being. *International Journal of Circumpolar Health*, 63(2), 140–144. doi: 10.3402/ijch.v63i2.17700

149 Siems, W. (1999). Improved antioxidative protection in winter swimmers. *Qjm*, 92(4), 193–198. doi: 10.1093/qjmed/92.4.193

150 *Living Philosophies*, 1931.

151 Shiota, M. N., Keltner, D., Mossman, A. (2007). The nature of awe: Elicitors, appraisals, and effects on self-concept. *Cognition & Emotion*, 21(5), 944–963. doi: 10.1080/02699930600923668

152 Matei, A. (2017, August 9). *Technology is changing our relationship with nature as we know it.* Retrieved from https://qz.com/1048433/technology-is-changing -our-relationship-with-nature-as-we-know-it/

153 O*man Forest Information and Data*. Retrieved from https://rainforests
.mongabay.com/deforestation/2000/Oman.htm

154 Flatt, M. (2015, July 16). *Nature and technology: friends or enemies?* Retrieved
from http://www.bbc.com/earth/story/20150703-can-nature-and-technology
-be-friends

155 Kahn, J. P. H., Weiss, T. (2017). The Importance of Children Interacting
with Big Nature. *Children, Youth and Environments*, 27(2), 7. doi: 10.7721/
chilyoutenvi.27.2.0007

156 University of Washington. (2017, November 15). *What counts as 'nature'? It all
depends*. ScienceDaily. Retrieved from www.sciencedaily.com
/releases/2017/11/171115124514.htm

157 Lymeus, F., Lindberg, P., Hartig, T. (2019). A natural meditation setting
improves compliance with mindfulness training. *Journal of Environmental
Psychology*, 64, 98–106. doi: 10.1016/j.jenvp.2019.05.008

158 Gamble, K. R., Howard, J. H., Howard, D. V. (2014). Not Just
Scenery: Viewing Nature Pictures Improves Executive Attention in
Older Adults. *Experimental Aging Research*, 40(5), 513–530. doi:
10.1080/0361073x.2014.956618. See also: Berto, R. (2005). Exposure
to restorative environments helps restore attentional capacity. *Journal of
Environmental Psychology*, 25(3), 249–259. doi: 10.1016/j.jenvp.2005.07.001

159 Kjellgren, A., Buhrkall, H. (2010). A comparison of the restorative effect of a
natural environment with that of a simulated natural environment. *Journal of
Environmental Psychology*, 30(4), 464–472. doi: 10.1016/j.jenvp.2010.01.011.
See also: Valtchanov, D., Barton, K. R., Ellard, C. (2010). Restorative Effects of
Virtual Nature Settings. *Cyberpsychology, Behavior, and Social Networking*, 13(5),
503–512. doi: 10.1089/cyber.2009.0308

160 Manaker, G. H. (1996). *Interior Plantscapes: Installation, maintenance, and
management* (3rd ed.). Prentice-Hall.

161 Cummings, B. E., Waring, M. S. (2019). Potted plants do not improve indoor
air quality: a review and analysis of reported VOC removal efficiencies. *Journal
of Exposure Science & Environmental Epidemiology*. 30, 253–261. doi: 10.1038/
s41370-019-0175-9

162 Bringslimark, T., Hartig, T., Patil, G. G. (2009). The psychological benefits
of indoor plants: A critical review of the experimental literature. *Journal of
Environmental Psychology*, 29(4), 422–433. doi: 10.1016/j.jenvp.2009.05.001

163 Watson, J. E. M., Venter, O., Lee, J., Jones, K. R., Robinson, J. G., Possingham, H. P., Allan, J. R. (2018). Protect the last of the wild. *Nature*, 563(7729), 27–30. doi: 10.1038/d41586-018-07183-6

164 Buxton, R. T., Mckenna, M. F., Mennitt, D., Fristrup, K., Crooks, K., Angeloni, L., Wittemyer, G. (2017). Noise pollution is pervasive in U.S. protected areas. *Science*, 356(6337), 531–533. doi: 10.1126/science.aah4783

165 National Park Service (2019, November 7). *Air Quality*. Retrieved from https://www.nps.gov/grsm/learn/nature/air-quality.htm

166 Pierno, T. (2017). Trash Talk. *National Parks*, 91(1).

167 Haigney, S. (2018, December 7). *How Stone Stacking Wreaks Havoc on National Parks*. Retrieved from https://www.newyorker.com/culture/rabbit-holes/people-are-stacking-too-many-stones

168 Peterson, D. (2000, October 1). *Bears And The "Blend In" Theory*. Retrieved from https://www.backpacker.com/stories/bears-and-the-34-blend-in-34-theory

169 Simon, G. L., Alagona, P. S. (2009). Beyond Leave No Trace. *Ethics, Place & Environment*, 12(1), 17–34. doi: 10.1080/13668790902753021

170 Patagonia. *Patagonia's Mission Statement*. Retrieved from https://www.patagonia.com/company-info.html

Made in the USA
Columbia, SC
04 September 2020